DR. SYDNEY'S

IGNORE YOUR TEETH and THEY'LL GO AWAY™

The Complete Guide to Gum Disease

SHELDON DOV SYDNEY, DDS

Board Certified and Associate Professor in Periodontics
University of Maryland School of Dentistry

DEVIDA PUBLICATIONS
Baltimore, Maryland

D1566195

OUTSTANDING REVIEWS

Ignore Your Teeth and They'll Go Away is the most professionally reviewed and recommended patient guide to gum disease ever written! Even gum specialists bought thousands of copies for their *own* patients to explain periodontal disease. Listed below are some of the many respected organizations' reviews of previous editions.

Journal of The American Dental Association

"Dr. Sydney's book is admirably suited to its intended audience... clear and concise... techniques described and illustrated so the patient can understand."

The American Library Association's Booklist

"Sydney, a professor at the University of Maryland School of Dentistry, is an authority on periodontal (gum) disease. His guide is precise and readily accessible to the general reader... works as an effective warning."

The British Dental Journal

"This book helps to reassure the public that it is possible to treat and save teeth. Should help to dispel much of the fear and ignorance which has shrouded periodontal disease and its treatment."

American Association for The Advancement of Science: Science Books and Films

"If you want to prevent or halt periodontal disease faithfully follow Sydney's advice. Sydney wonderfully reassures us as he guides readers step-by-step through each phase of treatment and even manages to take the fear out of the word "surgery"." Clearly described in non-technical terms."

Dentistry Today

The sequencing of chapters is logical with each chapter being set out in concise terms, especially the chapter plaque control, and the final chapter nicely answers many of the commonly asked questions."

The West Coast Review of Books

"Dr. Sydney demystifies what your periodontist does. Few books put me through changes. This one made me set up a dental appointment as soon as I could. I wish it had been available two teeth ago!"

New York State Dental Journal

"... provides the dental consumer with a clear, precise, well-written guide to the diagnosis and treatment of periodontal (gum) diseases and what to expect during and following periodontal and implant therapy."

The Journal of the New Jersey Dental Association

"Dr. Sydney's years of experience in periodontal practice and teaching as well as his ability to communicate are clearly demonstrated in this comprehensive, easy-to-read and understand guide."

New Hampshire Dental Society News

"Siding with practitioners who believe the patient should know what is going on, Sydney provides a step-by-step explanation of periodontal disease... admirable candor and clarity."

The Virginia Dental Journal "...Sydney has written first comprehensive guide to periodontal disease for the public, in simple language, easy for the layman to understand. The author unravels fact from myth. The choice is clear to the patient. Ignore your teeth and they'll go away, but heed the timely information in this book and you can enjoy your teeth for a lifetime."

IGNORE YOUR TEETH AND THEY'LL GO AWAY
The Complete Guide to Gum Disease

4th Edition

Library of Congress Control Number: 2015913568

ISBN 978-0-9968121-0-8

e-ISBN 978-0-9968121-1-5

Copyright © 1982 First Edition, 1988 Second Edition,
1998 Third Edition, 2016 Fourth Edition
by Sheldon Dov Sydney, DDS. All rights reserved.

Publisher: Devida Pubications
Author: Dr. Sheldon Dov Sydney
Managing Editor: Guy Sydney EMT-P
Scientific Consultant: Professor Phillip Dowell
Design and Production: Estee Art&Design
Art Direction: Esther Weiser Kreisman
Production Assistant: Yonit Nir
Illustrator: S. Sommer
Copy Editing: Deborah Sydney BA, MA
Director of Marketing: Sharan Kushner
Proofreading: Sarita and Dan Sragow

DISCLAIMER

This book is a general reference and information guide only, designed to help the reader make informed decisions regarding periodontal health and dental implants. It is not intended as dental treatment manual or advice for any particular individual's oral and/or periodontal problems. Prior to undertaking any treatment including those subjects either discussed or suggested in this book, the reader should consult with a periodontal specialist or experienced dentist with training in the diagnosis and treatment of periodontal diseases and dental implants. Neither of the author nor the publisher shall be liable or responsible for any injury, or damage allegedly arising from any information or suggestions in this book

Devida Publications
205 John Eager Court, Baltimore, Maryland 21208
For information regarding sales and promotions: e-mail: ignoreyourteeth@devida.com

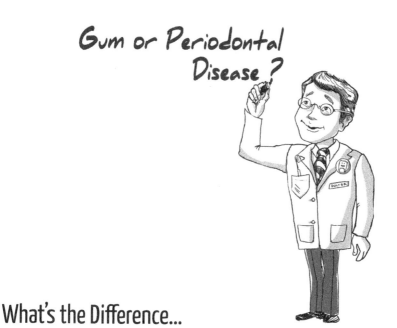

Gum or Periodontal Disease ?

What's the Difference...

When using the expression *gum disease* people are actually referring to a type of periodontal disease. The word periodontal is derived from the Latin "peri" for around and "odont" for tooth. Periodontal identifies the location of those diseases and conditions affecting the structures surrounding and supporting the teeth. The preference for the term periodontal disease is found in every major dental textbook as well as in communications between health professionals.

However, since the familiar signs of periodontal disease appear in the gums, the term gum disease has become the layman's more widely recognized name. It was subsequently selected as the subtitle of this book. In order however to integrate readers' familiarity with the correct terminology, references to both gum disease and periodontal disease are used interchangeably to identify the same disease entities.

IGNORE YOUR TEETH

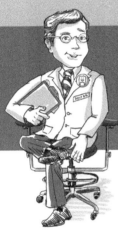

CONTENTS

PART I Basic Understandings

PART II Evaluation

and THEY'LL GO AWAY™

The Complete Guide to Gum Disease

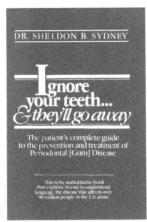
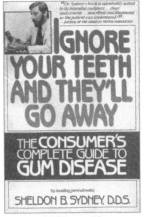
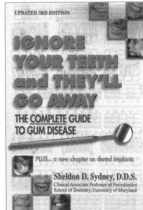

1st Edition 1982   *2nd Edition 1988*   *3rd Edition 1998*

Introduction to the Fourth Edition
The Tradition Continues

Looking back at the previous three editions' covers, I can't help but think of the thousands of consumers, patients and colleagues over the last 30 years who have depended on *Ignore Your Teeth and They'll Go Away* as the premier guide for making informed decisions regarding care of their gums.

The significant progress that has emerged since the last edition in the treatment of gum disease and dental implants has been included. New terminology and expressions officially adopted by the profession have been chosen where there is variance with previous editions. I've also introduced a new feature called "From my files" containing real patient histories. Of course, their true identities have been altered to protect their privacy. As always, the reader can be assured that all procedures and therapies discussed in this book have been scrupulously evaluated and are established, predictable treatments based on firm scientific principles. Alternative or experimental approaches, when discussed, are clearly identified as such.

Despite the availability of many successful treatment options, nearly 80% the world's adults are still affected by gum disease; 44% may have lost their teeth by the age of 65. But the most alarming of all statistics is that half of all school children have gingivitis, the first stage periodontal disease.

The solution is in your hands. As an informed consumer/patient you can save your own teeth and your families' teeth from the ravages of gum disease. To begin with, if you have any of the warning signs of gum disease (see opening page of Chapter 3) seek immediate professional advice from your dentist or periodontist, an expert in the diagnosis and treatment of gum disease and the placement of dental implants. If you are symptom-free, ask your dentist for periodontal evaluation during regular checkups to ensure no disease is present. In addition, make use of this book to learn as much as possible about gum disease. Discover how to get started, diagnosed and treated. Find out why some individuals are more susceptible than others, and get the answers to the most commonly asked questions. But most importantly, take to heart the chapter on prevention. There you will acquire the basic techniques of controlling the cause of gum disease: bacterial plaque.

Ignore your teeth and they'll go away? Sure, it's funny, just like it was when I first titled this book in 1982, but unfortunately, it's also true! The fact that you are reading this guide right now, means you have already decided that the health of your gums is no laughing matter. And that is a good start. Because the more you understand about gum disease, the better are your chances of keeping your teeth for a lifetime of healthy, beautiful smiles.

Sheldon Dov Sydney

Acknowledgments

To the greatest of parents, the late Dr. Elmer L. Sydney, and Mrs. Fern Sydney Swerdlin. With the passing of time, my appreciation for all they have done for me and the pride in being their son only deepens. My children, Deborah, David, Aviva, Michal and Guy have rewarded me with many reasons to feel blessed. And of course, the unbelievable good fortune in having married Rachel. Her unwavering support, uncanny intuitiveness and unshakable love can never be measured.

To colleagues and mentors: Dr. Gerald Bowers, former Executive Director the American Board of Periodontology; Dr. John Bergquist Past Chairman Department of Periodontology at the University of Maryland; Dr. Shalom Sussman, former District President and my sponsor to the International College of Dentists; Dr. Michael Fritz, Editor Emeritus, *Journal of Periodontology*; and Dr. Mel Kushner, Past President Maryland Board of Dental Examiners.

Special note of appreciation to: Sharan Kushner, Marketing Director, for her enthusiasm, tenacity and loyalty to Devida projects; Prof. Phillip Dowell, Past President of the British Society of Periodontology, for his role as scientific consultant and manuscript reviewer; and Managing Editor Guy Sydney, who inspired and encouraged me to write this edition, was involved in every aspect of its preparation, and continues his contributions in the post-production phase even while attending medical school.

Last, but not least, I would like to thank my patients and postgraduate students who, for more than 30 years, have never failed to provide me with the inspiration, challenge and fulfillment to work in this wonderful profession.

PART I
Basic Understandings

1

A Journey Back in Time

How History
has Recorded
Man's Eternal
Battle with Gum
Disorders

Discoveries from Ancient Civilizations

Studies of preserved skulls have established that periodontal (gum) diseases existed in prehistoric times. Recorded history has documented a surprising awareness of periodontal disease throughout the ages.

Embalmed Egyptian mummies from four thousand years ago reveal that periodontal disease was common among the Pharaohs. Ancient papyri also contain significant references to gum problems and suggestions for treatment.

The Sumerians (3000 BCE) attempted to practice dental hygiene. Excavations in Mesopotamia have discovered exquisitely designed golden toothpicks used for removing food deposits between the teeth. Later in history, a clay tablet found from the Babylonian and Assyrian periods, revealed that these people suffered from periodontal disease. The clay tablet tells of the need to treat gum problems with massage combined with herbal medicine.

In 2500 BCE, Hwang-Fi wrote the oldest known Chinese medical work which included extensive discussion of oral diseases. He divided them into three types: inflammation, diseases of soft tissues of the teeth and tooth decay. He called these three divisions Fong

Ya, Ya Kon and Chong Ya, respectively. His work includes accurate descriptions of gum inflammations, abscesses and ulcerations, which would be perfectly recognizable today. He describes one condition in this way: "The gingivae are pale or violet red, hard and lumpy, sometimes bleeding, and the toothache is continuous."

The early Hebrews recognized the importance of oral hygiene. Many conditions of the teeth and gums are described in Talmudic writings. A specimen from the ancient Phoenician civilization shows an attempt at wire splinting to stabilize teeth loosened by periodontal disease (Fig. 1-1).

As early as the time of Hippocrates (460-335 BCE) it was known that inflammation of the gums could be caused by accumulations of tartar or calculus, and that bleeding gums frequently occurred in advanced cases of periodontal disease.

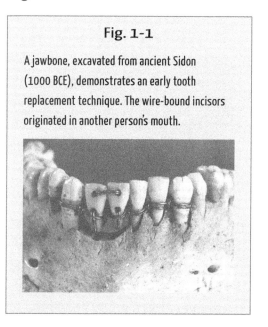

Fig. 1-1

A jawbone, excavated from ancient Sidon (1000 BCE), demonstrates an early tooth replacement technique. The wire-bound incisors originated in another person's mouth.

Roman Times In the first century, the Roman Lulus Cornelius Celsus wrote about diseases affecting the soft tissues of the mouth. He prescribed: "If the gums separate from the teeth, it is beneficial to chew unripe pears and apples and keep their juices in the mouth." He also described teeth loosened by deterioration of the gums, and recommended treating them by touching the gums lightly with a red-hot iron, and then rubbing them with honey and/or narcotics.

Other ancient writers suggested medications ranging from opium, oil of roses and honey, to astringent mouth washes, dentifrice powders, and even counterirritants in treating gum disease.

Avicenna (980-1037 BCE) was probably the earliest scientist to explore the importance of a proper bite in periodontal disease. He wrote about filing elongated teeth to adjust the bite.

About the same time, Albucasis (936-1013 BCE) analyzed the need to care for the tooth-supporting structures, and recognized the importance of removing tartar. With a little modernization of language, his writings might be found in a twentieth-century dental text. He wrote: "Sometimes on the surface of the teeth, both inside and outside, as well as under the gums, are deposited rough scales of ugly appearance and black, green or yellow in color. This corruption is communicated to the gums, and so the teeth are, in the process of time, denuded. It is necessary for thee to lay the patient's head upon thy lap and to scrape the teeth and molars, on which are observed either true incrustations, or something similar to sand, and this until nothing more remains of such substance..."

Perilous Sea Travels As civilization advanced, man began to travel. Sailors often suffered from extreme vitamin deficiency due to the long and sometimes miscalculated trips between shores. As a result, they developed gum-related vitamin C deficiency known as scurvy, the occupational disease of the time. Lost at sea, many times without supplies and lacking preservatives, the sailors hunted and killed rats for food.

Scurvy, revealed its most devastating effects in the jawbone, loosening teeth and causing severe overgrowth of bleeding gums. In great pain, the sailors would slash each other's gums in order to reduce the pressure from this infection.

Names Worth Remembering

What You See is What You Get When Anton van Leeuwenhoek (1632-1723) invented the microscope, he was certainly unaware that over two hundred years later, the little creatures he found and described through his lens (taken from the saliva of his own mouth) would become the bacterial foundation for the study of periodontal disease. What he saw then for the first time were plaque-forming germs or bacteria!

Pierre Fauchard   It was with his book published in 1728, "The Surgeon Dentist – a Treatise on Teeth," that Pierre Fauchard (Fig. 1-3) emerged as the father of modern dentistry.

The Frenchman wrote on a broad range of dental subjects from dental chairs to dentures. In particular, his writings on pyorrhea (an old name for gum disease) were so often quoted that for a time it was called "Fauchard's Disease."

Fig. 1-2

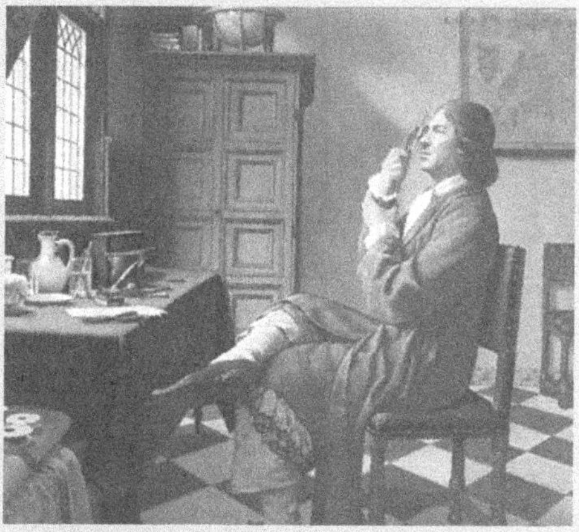

In this painting, Anton van Leeuwenhoek (1632 to 1723) is seen peeking through the first rudimentary microscope.

John Hunter   England's John Hunter, a physician and surgeon, expanded current knowledge of teeth and gums with his work "The Natural History of the Human Teeth" published in 1778. In this now classic text, Hunter accurately described how gum disease began at the gum edge, working its way down the root and eventually destroying the connection of the tooth to the bone.

Dr. Riggs' Special Place in History   In the United States, Dr. John M. Riggs (1810-1885) of Hartford, Connecticut probably did more than any other individual to establish the basis of modern periodontics with his use of specific instruments for the treatment of gum disease.

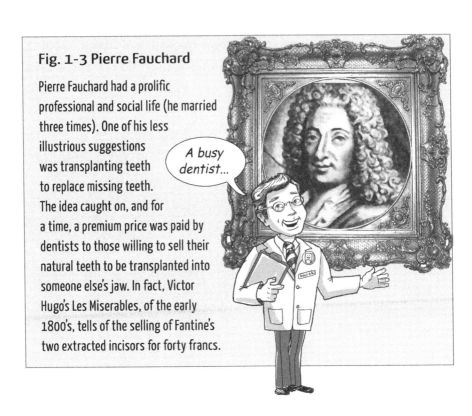

Fig. 1-3 Pierre Fauchard

Pierre Fauchard had a prolific professional and social life (he married three times). One of his less illustrious suggestions was transplanting teeth to replace missing teeth. The idea caught on, and for a time, a premium price was paid by dentists to those willing to sell their natural teeth to be transplanted into someone else's jaw. In fact, Victor Hugo's Les Miserables, of the early 1800's, tells of the selling of Fantine's two extracted incisors for forty francs.

A busy dentist...

He was a frequent lecturer and author who encouraged many dentists to adopt his methods. Though he originally began his education as a priest and later attended medical school, Dr. Riggs eventually chose dentistry and specifically periodontics as a career. Some of his basic techniques still have applications in today's modern therapy.

Dr. John Riggs (Fig. 1-4) was a participant in one of the most dramatic advances in medicine. His colleague and friend, Dr. Horace Wells, discovered anesthesia, after seeing a circus show where "laughing gas" or nitrous oxide was demonstrated. Being inquisitive and also suffering from a toothache too advanced even for Dr. Riggs' renowned methods, Dr. Wells asked Riggs to remove the tooth, but only after administering the gas. In December of 1844, having successfully removed the offending tooth with no pain, Riggs obtained the distinction of performing the first surgical procedure with the aid of anesthesia anywhere in the world.

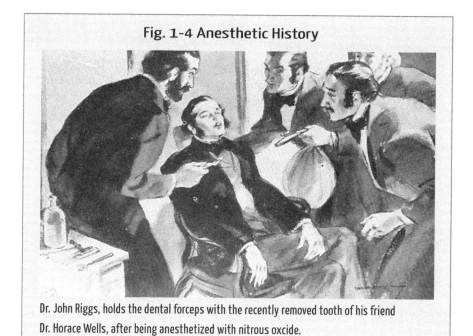

Fig. 1-4 Anesthetic History

Dr. John Riggs, holds the dental forceps with the recently removed tooth of his friend Dr. Horace Wells, after being anesthetized with nitrous oxide.

Dental Education

Early on, dentistry was taught as an apprenticeship because no formal dental colleges existed. Chapin Harris, a physician, became interested in dentistry and traveled throughout the southern United States practicing dentistry and medicine. He moved to Baltimore and studied with Horace Hayden, a dentist who lectured to medical students at the University of Baltimore.

Harris and Hayden hoped to develop a department of dentistry in the university's medical school, but were unable to gain acceptance by the faculty. They petitioned the State of Maryland for a charter, and in 1840 the Baltimore College of Dental Surgery (Fig. 1-5) became the first dental college in the world with the authority to award the degree D.D.S. (Doctor of Dental Surgery). Dr. F. H. Rehwinkel, a German physician, became interested in dentistry and

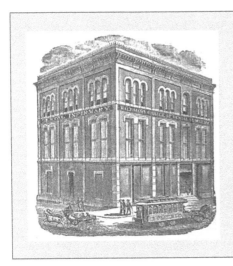

Fig. 1-5

World's First Dental School

The first dental school in the world opened its doors as the Baltimore College of Dental Surgery in Baltimore, Maryland in 1840 . The dental school, now part of the University of Maryland complex, has continued to train dentists and dental specialists from throughout the United States as well as the rest of the world.

graduated from the Maryland dental school in 1854. He is credited with first using the term "pyorrhea" to describe gum disease in a paper presented in August 1877.

The Specialty of Periodontics   Soon the need developed for formalized, advanced education beyond the basic dental degree, for dentists who could provide specialized skills to patients suffering from diseases of the gums and tooth-supporting structures. The specialty that emerged to meet this need would be known as periodontics or periodontology, and the specialist in these diseases, a periodontist. In 1914, the first professional society devoted exclusively to periodontal disease as a specialty, the American Academy of Periodontology (AAP), was founded.

Over the ensuing years, periodontal specialty societies were established throughout the world and have done much to advance the periodontal health of the public and promote excellence in the practice of periodontics. This includes the assurance of quality specialty programs and continuing education opportunities for dentists interested in studying periodontics.

The local periodontal specialist society in your area (depending on local laws and customs) will usually be the principal authority on all matters dealing with periodontics for health care providers and consumers. In addition, these societies represent the dental professionals specializing in the prevention, diagnosis and treatment of periodontal diseases, and the placement and treatment of dental implants. For a listing of national and regional periodontal societies refer to the Part IV, Appendix, Finding a Periodontist.

Dramatic advances continue to be made by dedicated researchers and clinicians in our understanding of gum diseases, leading to an ever-increasing range of predictable therapies. However, it should be clear by now, that today's discoveries have not developed in a vacuum, but are built on the shoulders of giants from a remarkable history.

2

The Jaw Bone's Connected to the...

The Anatomy of a
Healthy Mouth

The Teeth

Each tooth is unique in size, shape and function. Molars, for example, have large, wide biting surfaces and two or three roots that are utilized for the heavy biting pressures necessary to emulsify the food. Incisors, on the other hand, are shaped for their shearing ability, because they tear the food into smaller pieces for the molars to chew.

Teeth grow out of sockets formed from the upper and lower jaw bones called alveolar bone, which surround the roots of the teeth and provide support during chewing.

The tooth, however, does not fit exactly within the socket. A slight space between tooth and bone contains fibrous threads of tissue that hold the tooth to the bone and provide a shock-absorbing layer permitting slight movement under pressure. These highly specialized fiber attachments are called the periodontal ligaments. Alongside the periodontal ligaments pass blood vessels that act as conduits for nutrition and nerves that carry signals from the brain. The signals transfer information relative to the exact position of the teeth and jaws, to and from the brain to the tongue and cheek during chewing and speech.

Ignore Your Teeth and They'll Go Away

Fig. 2-1 The Teeth

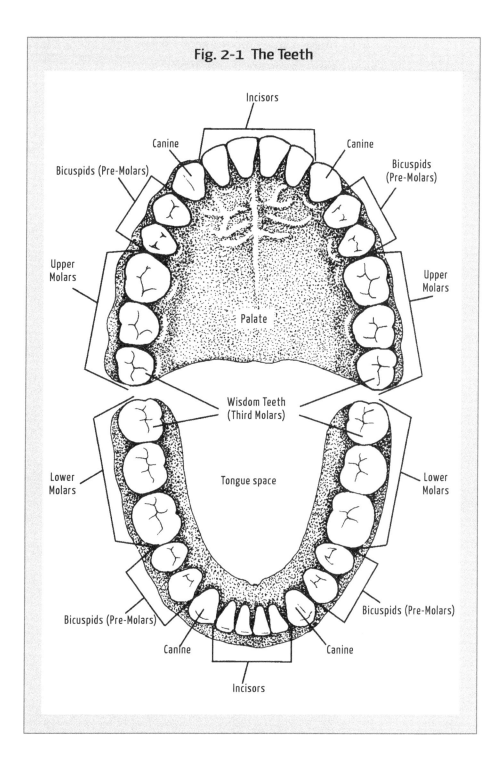

Incisors

Canine

Canine

Bicuspids (Pre-Molars)

Bicuspids (Pre-Molars)

Upper Molars

Upper Molars

Palate

Wisdom Teeth (Third Molars)

Lower Molars

Lower Molars

Tongue space

Bicuspids (Pre-Molars)

Bicuspids (Pre-Molars)

Canine

Canine

Incisors

Periodontal ligaments are embedded in a special root surface called the cementum. The cementum has a porous surface that facilitates adherence to the periodontal ligament.

Finally, the enamel is the hard, protective outer layer covering the exposed portion of the tooth above the gum line, and the first defense against cavities. Inside the body of the tooth is found the dental pulp. Within it are the nerves, blood vessels and other life-supporting mechanisms that keep the interior of the tooth healthy.

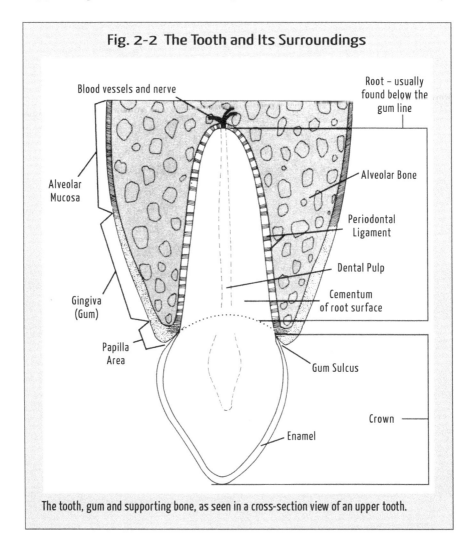

Fig. 2-2 The Tooth and Its Surroundings

Blood vessels and nerve

Root – usually found below the gum line

Alveolar Mucosa

Alveolar Bone

Periodontal Ligament

Dental Pulp

Gingiva (Gum)

Cementum of root surface

Papilla Area

Gum Sulcus

Crown

Enamel

The tooth, gum and supporting bone, as seen in a cross-section view of an upper tooth.

Ignore Your Teeth and They'll Go Away

The Gums (Gingiva)

Several different tissues comprise what we know as "gums." The technical name is gingiva and includes the tissues that extend from the jaws to the necks of the teeth.

The gingiva is the coral-pink tissue, which blankets the area of the root and bone, providing important protection for these underlying structures.

Healthy gums form an attractive smile.

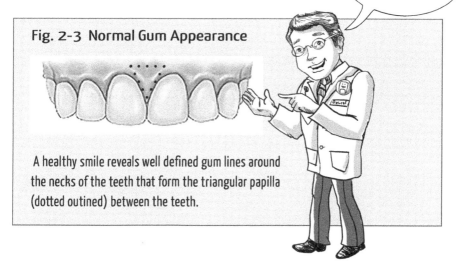

Fig. 2-3 Normal Gum Appearance

A healthy smile reveals well defined gum lines around the necks of the teeth that form the triangular papilla (dotted outlined) between the teeth.

The triangular shaped papilla is an extension of the gingiva filling the space between the teeth (Fig. 2-3). In general, the presence of healthy papillae between the teeth contributes substantially to an attractive looking smile.

Around the neck of each tooth, the gingiva has a fold of tissue that forms a small v-shaped groove called the sulcus. The sulcus is where most periodontal disease starts. Usually the gum sulcus is slightly over a millimeter or two in depth, or about one tenth of an inch.Under healthy conditions, the sulcus is tightly adapted to the tooth and relatively free of contaminants.

Continuing past the gingiva into the furrow where the lip and jawbone meet is the alveolar mucosa. This thin, almost transparent tissue is a direct continuation of the gingiva, although technically not gingiva. The alveolar mucosa which covers the jawbone (alveolar bone) has a glistening appearance, which usually contrasts sharply with the leathery and pale texture of the gingiva.

Ignore Your Teeth and They'll Go Away

3

Periodontal Diseases

From Normal Teeth
to Toothless Gums

Warning Signs of Periodontal (Gum) Disease

- Bleeding gums when you brush your teeth
- Red, swollen or tender gums
- Bad breath (halitosis)
- Gums that have shrunk away from your teeth
- Any change in the way your teeth come together
- Any change in the way your partial dentures fit
- Pus between your teeth and gums when you press them
- Loose or separated permanent teeth

Despite these warning signs, periodontal disease affects more than 75% of all adults worldwide. How this disease can work so insidiously and destructively is a subject worthy of further understanding.

Bacterial Plaque

Without question, the number one cause of periodontal or gum disease is bacterial plaque, sometimes referred to as biofilm because it is composed of biologically active elements. Plaque is a thin, colorless, sticky substance found on tooth surfaces.

How is plaque formed? Within a few minutes after a tooth has been completely cleaned, the process of plaque formation begins. Bacteria (Fig. 3-1) in the mouth begins collecting either directly on the surface of the teeth or on what is called the pellicle, which is an intervening, imperceptible coating formed on the teeth from proteins in the saliva. (Remember the important discovery of Anton van Leeuwenhoek described in Chapter 1?).

Additional layers of deposits and bacteria adhere to and expand

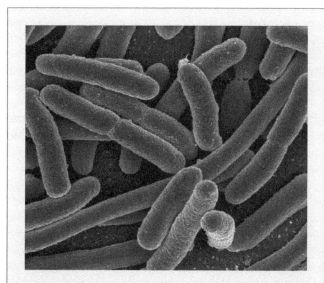

Fig. 3-1 Bacteria

In this high-powered microscopic view, a single type of bacteria is seen. However more than 500 different bacteria have been found to inhabit the human mouth. The more destructive varieties can cause great damage to the gums and tooth-supporting bones.

the plaque surface, so that within hours after teeth have been thoroughly cleaned, measurable amounts of plaque can be detected. The rate of plaque accumulation varies in different individuals and on different teeth in a particular person.

Left completely alone with no effort to remove it, plaque will reach a maximum thickness of a soft white material in about thirty days. During the course of the build-up, the types of bacteria become more virulent. If allowed to continue unabated, plaque bacteria will release poisons or toxins that stimulate the destructive series of events leading to gum disease.

Calculus (Tartar) Traces of mineral salts found in saliva combine with the plaque to form a hard, porous, calcified deposit on the teeth called calculus, more commonly known as tartar. Chemically speaking, calculus is a cousin of boiler scale, and is no more desirable in your mouth than clogged pipes in your home, as it provides an attractive surface for plaque accumulation.

The Battle For Superiority

How We React to Plaque When you catch a cold, it is not actually the invading cold virus that causes you to have the fever, headaches, sniffles and sneezing. Those symptoms are all part of the body's response to the invading virus. Our understanding of this phenomenon comes by way of the study of microbiology (germs) and immunology (the human defensive systems). The battle between the invading bacterial plaque and the defense devices of one's own body is central to understanding the destructive results of periodontal disease.

When gum tissue cells recognize that they are in contact with potentially destructive bacterial plaque or its poisons, the body's protective system sends out blood, rich in defensive equipment, to fight the invaders. The battle goes on as the bacteria attempt to gain superiority in numbers and strength, while the immune system fights back vigorously with its own defensive mechanisms. The battle can lead to red and swollen gum tissue and the beginning of a destructive disease cycle.

Host Response Today, the term host response is used to describe the unique nature of each human or host to mount an effective defense to infection. Regarding periodontal disease, we have discovered many aspects of the host response that influence an individual's reaction to plaque and its toxins.

Unfortunately, there is still much we do not understand. In the future, this ever-expanding field is likely to provide us with new basic tools with which to treat or prevent disease. For now, we can summarize this subject by saying that if an individual has a good host response, the damage caused by the gum diseases will likely be less destructive than in an individual with a poor host response.

Is anyone listening?

Bleeding Gums

How is it so many esthetic-minded, health conscious, intelligent people allow their gums to bleed day in and day out without the slightest concern? Why is there so little anxiety about gum bleeding? Bleeding indicates that there is an invasion of bacteria, inflammation and INFECTION, warning of danger to the gums, just as infection would be a serious concern elsewhere in the body.

There is no question that blood oozing from the ear or coughed-up would send most of us running immediately to a professional for help. Why? Because we know bleeding always signifies something is wrong! Bleeding in the mouth however, has been considered "normal" for so long that this important early warning sign is being ignored (remember the title of this book?). A periodontist or other dental professional must evaluate any amount of bleeding in the mouth.

Types of Periodontal Diseases

There are different types of periodontal disease. The discussion below refers to the major forms caused by plaque, and those most likely to be treated by your therapist.

Gingivitis

Gingivitis, an early gum infection, is a reversible disease characterized by tenderness, swelling, and most importantly, bleeding of the gum tissue. In the United States, a majority of youngsters over the age of thirteen already have gingivitis! The normal, healthy pink color darkens from the increase in blood volume, and goes through various shades of red. In more advanced cases, the gums may appear reddish-blue. Gingivitis usually begins gradually and progresses as symptoms become more prominent. It can, however, be a fluctuating disease. For example, inflamed areas develop and then become normal, only for inflammation to reappear at a later date. Bad breath, which frequently accompanies periodontal diseases, may first develop during gingivitis.

The Periodontal Pocket

If plaque accumulation did no more than cause irritation or gingivitis, we might not be so concerned. Unfortunately, because most bleeding is ignored, the advantage is lost of detecting early signs of periodontal disease and receiving prompt and relatively simple care. If the disease progresses, serious consequences can develop.

As noted earlier, the gum reacts to plaque with swelling and inflammation. This condition permits the plaque to approach the normally well-adapted crevice or sulcus between the gingiva and tooth. The infection spreads into the attachment causing the gum to separate from the tooth.

With the gum seal broken, more plaque can bury itself within the newly enlarged gum space. The space created by this separation is called a periodontal pocket (Fig. 3-2) and represents the critical pathologic entity of periodontal disease. In general, it is the comparative measurement of these pockets that reveals the extent and seriousness of periodontal disease.

Chronic Periodontitis

As the gum infection advances along the root, the pocket deepens with destruction of bone and attaching fibers. This condition is called periodontitis and the most common type is known as chronic periodontitis. The disease slowly progresses over time and is further distinguished by its severity, i.e. early, moderate or severe periodontitis (Fig. 3-3) as well as whether it affects a few teeth (local) or most of the teeth in the mouth (general).

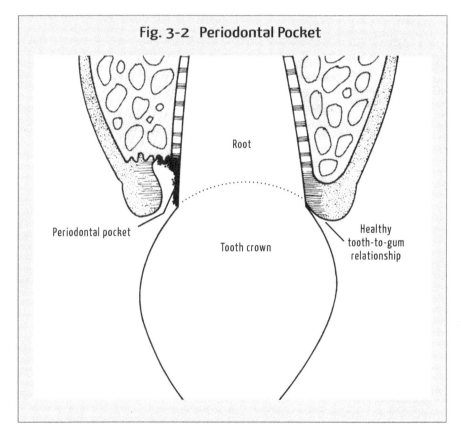

Fig. 3-2 Periodontal Pocket

Root

Periodontal pocket

Tooth crown

Healthy
tooth-to-gum
relationship

Periodontitis has been referred to as pyorrhea, which literally means "pus flow." Pus can develop as supporting bone is destroyed and interacts with the infected gum tissue, usually in the latter stages of the disease. Sometimes so much support is destroyed that the teeth become loose. Periodontitis is serious business. Left untreated, periodontitis has the potential to continue for many years as a chronic, progressive infection, and a true threat to the survival of the teeth.

Aggressive Periodontitis

A very destructive type of periodontal disease, less common than chronic periodontitis, is known as aggressive periodontitis (AgP). Individuals with aggressive periodontitis demonstrate significant and rapid bone loss around their teeth. The disease is particularly disturbing as it is often diagnosed in children and young adults. It can first appear around the time of puberty or even earlier, although it is also diagnosed later in life. A peculiar characteristic often seen with AgP is that destruction of underlying bone can be extensive even though there is only a surprisingly small amount of plaque in the mouth.

As in the case of chronic periodontitis, this disease can affect a few isolated teeth or the entire mouth. The local type seems to be more self-limiting, while the general form is often more extensive and may be difficult to manage.

AgP patients do not always respond well to routine periodontal therapy. Some systemic diseases or altered mechanisms of the body are thought to contribute to the unpredictability and difficulty in treating AgP. The influence of defective cells in the body's defense mechanism have been suggested as one explanation. Also, this type of periodontal disease is frequently found among family members, supporting the likelihood of a genetic predisposition to AgP.

Gum Recession and Exposed Roots

Occasionally gum tissues recede along with the loss of bone, especially on the front root surfaces of the teeth where the bone is

Fig. 3-3 Progress of Periodontal Diseases

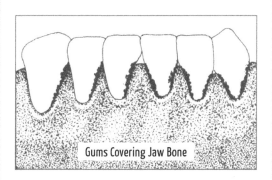

Gums Covering Jaw Bone

Gingivitis

Plaque and tartar accumulate along the gum lines and the necks of the teeth. Gums swell and begin to show evidence of bleeding. Gums are no longer well adapted to the tooth and the gum space (sulcus) may be widen.

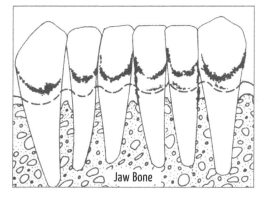

Jaw Bone

Early to Moderate Periodontitis

(gum tissues not drawn in) Plaque advances below the gum line along with the beginning of pocket formation. Early bone loss is noted which may be accompanied by recession of the gums (dotted line).

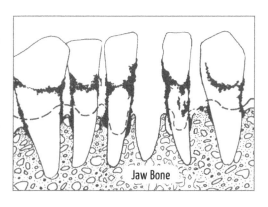

Jaw Bone

Severe Periodontitis and Tooth Loss

Teeth become loose, plaque and tartar advance down the root surfaces. The gum line may continue to recede. Bone is destroyed leaving deep defects and pockets with infection. Pus and abscess formation often occur along with the loss of teeth.

thin and the roots tend to bulge. Often accompanying the esthetic defect is temperature sensitivity resulting from root exposure. Heavy tooth brushing can cause certain kinds of recession without inflammation being present.

Implant Related Gum and Periodontal Diseases

See Implant Chapter.

4

Other Gum Problems

Less Well-known Mouth Ailments

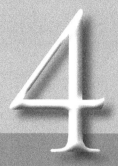

Gums Affected by other Conditions

Many conditions affect the mouth and gums, in addition to the diseases discussed in the previous chapter, which are not strictly members of the gingivitis or periodontitis categories. Reviewed in this chapter are other gum problems one might encounter.

Canker Sores

Small, white ulcerated areas found on the inside of the lips and mouth are usually canker sores or apthous ulcers. They are painful, especially when eating spicy foods, and last about ten days. While the cause has not been determined conclusively, some hypotheses include stress, nutritional, vitamin deficiency and allergy. Anesthetic creams placed directly on the sores are generally helpful until the symptoms subside. Canker sores are the most common kinds of lesions found in the mouth that cause patients to come to the dentist. They are however harmless.

Injuries to Gum Tissue

Many instances of accidental injury to the gum tissues have been reported in dental literature. Cuts in the gums are caused by unintentional scratching with fingernails as well as the improper use of dental floss, toothpicks and hard toothbrushes. The unjustified custom of placing aspirin tablets directly on painful gums has led to serious chemical burns. Also scalding soups and drinks, pizza or other hot and spicy foods can leave very sore blisters on gums, lips and the roof of the mouth.

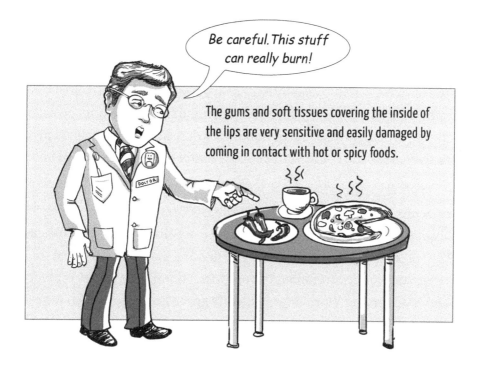

Abscess (Gum Boil)

An abscess (gum boil) is a collection of infected gum and sometimes bone tissue resulting in the formation of pus. It can cause pain. These isolated lesions usually develop from infection underneath the gum tissue within pre-existing periodontal pockets. Abscesses may also occur in healthy gums as a result of trapped food or foreign matter such as broken toothpicks.

Primary Oral Herpes

One of the few confirmed contagious gum diseases is primary oral herpes or acute herpetic gingivostomatitis. It generally lasts from a week to ten days. Frequently seen in children, it is caused by a virus. Symptoms include painful white and red sores in the gum area that may spread to the lips and throat. This disease is generally associated with a fever. Primary herpes is not the same virus that causes genital herpes, which results from sexual contact.

Necrotizing Diseases

The term necrotizing usually implies aggressive and rapid destruction of human tissues. These necrotizing gum diseases are not typical of the types of gingivitis and periodontitis described in the last chapter, as they generally begin with signs of tissue destruction and pain.

Acute Necrotizing Ulcerative Gingivitis (Trench Mouth) Trench mouth or acute necrotizing ulcerative gingivitis, sometimes known by its abbreviation ANUG, is characterized by a painful infection that can last as long as several weeks. This disease may also manifest as a recurring condition leading to bone loss. The widespread prevalence of ANUG among World War I soldiers gave rise to the trench mouth name. The condition however was even recognized in the fourth century during the Greek empire. Xenophon described fighters of the time were affected by "sore mouths and foul-smelling breath".

Though long considered to be contagious, more recent research has proved that this is not the case. Latest evidence suggests specific bacteria, plaque, stress, smoking and poor nutrition are associated with this disease.

Necrotizing Periodontitis A more advanced and destructive type of necrotizing gum disease is called necrotizing periodontitis, characterized by significant destruction of the supporting bone.

This disease is often associated with immune-deficient individuals such as those suffering from HIV infection. There is debate whether the two necrotizing diseases are actually one in the same disease.

Changes in Gum Color

A change in gum color can result from the absorption of certain heavy metals. Arsenic and mercury, for example, can produce a black line that follows the shape of the gum margin. Lead in the blood results in a bluish-red or deep purple line along the gum margin, while silver produces a bluish-gray discoloration throughout the membranes of the mouth.

Medicines such as minocycline, frequently used in acne therapy, are known to produce a black appearance to the gums. Alteration in gum color may also be caused by underlying medical problems. Addison's disease, for example, which is signified by a deficiency in a specialized hormone, may produce isolated black or brown patches on the gums. Smoking is also known to affect the appearance of the oral tissues by causing brownish stains or patches along the gums.

Swollen Gums

Puffy or swollen gums may be caused by conditions other than gum disease. Drugs used to prevent seizures, and certain heart medications, for example, can cause the gums to become puffy. In addition, there are numerous diseases whose secondary effects include gum swelling such as certain forms of anemia and leukemia. Therefore, should you have any signs of gum overgrowth, it is important that your mouth be examined by a dental professional.

Pericoronitis: Painful Gums Over Wisdom Teeth

Pericoronitis is a relatively common occurrence usually resulting when gum tissue grows over wisdom teeth (especially those that are not fully erupted) and becomes swollen and painful. Biting on the enlarged gums exacerbates this condition. Treatment involves either removal of the tooth, or treatment of the affected gum.

Skin Diseases

There are various skin diseases that also affect the soft tissues of the mouth. Some involve a local response to a specific allergy, while others can represent a generalized skin problem with complicating oral symptoms, such as psoriasis. A periodontist is trained to recognize these diseases and will in many cases, work with a skin specialist (dermatologist) to treat the problem.

Growths

Tumors or growths, both benign and malignant (cancerous), occur in the mouth and gum tissues. A trained professional is the only one who can evaluate if a growth is serious or not. A sample or biopsy of the suspected lesion may be required to confirm the diagnosis.

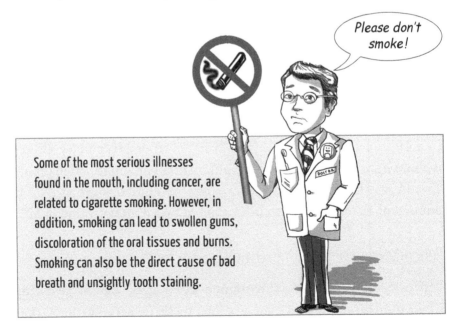

Please don't smoke!

Some of the most serious illnesses found in the mouth, including cancer, are related to cigarette smoking. However, in addition, smoking can lead to swollen gums, discoloration of the oral tissues and burns. Smoking can also be the direct cause of bad breath and unsightly tooth staining.

Bad Breath

Bad breath, or its technical term halitosis, can result from poor dental health habits and often a sign of both gingivitis and periodontitis. Bad breath can also result from other oral diseases and infections. In addition to problems stemming from the mouth, bad breath may be related to respiratory tract infections such as pneumonia or bronchitis, chronic sinus infections, postnasal drip, diabetes, chronic acid reflux, and liver or kidney problems.

PART II
Evaluation

5

A Visit to the Periodontist

What to Expect

Who is this Stranger, the Periodontist?

Most patients are referred for consultation by their dentists, friends or physicians. This is the moment when they may hear the word "periodontist" for the first time, and are confronted with the possibility that they have a disease requiring attention by a specialist.

The fact that periodontal disease does not usually cause pain, further mystifies the patient who generally associates disease with discomfort or other annoying symptoms. Along with this natural concern is a phenomenon of great anticipation resulting from second-hand "gum treatment experiences," related to the patient as soon as periodontal disease is brought up in casual conversation.

The Training of a Periodontist To begin with, all dentists learn the same basic dental studies and perform a wide variety of clinical procedures on patients, as required by the national or regional educational authorities. In North American dental schools, students first obtain an undergraduate degree from college or university. This is followed by four years of dental school, after which a dentist will receive either a D.D.S. (Doctor of Dental Surgery), or a D.M.D. (Doctor of Dental Medicine). Both of these degrees are identical in regard to the type of education and qualifications as a dentist. In Europe and other parts of the world, students begin dental studies directly out of high school and these programs take up to six years to complete and receive a dental degree.

A qualified dentist, if accepted, then attends an approved specialty program, which requires at least an additional three years of training, principally in the study of periodontal disease and dental implants.

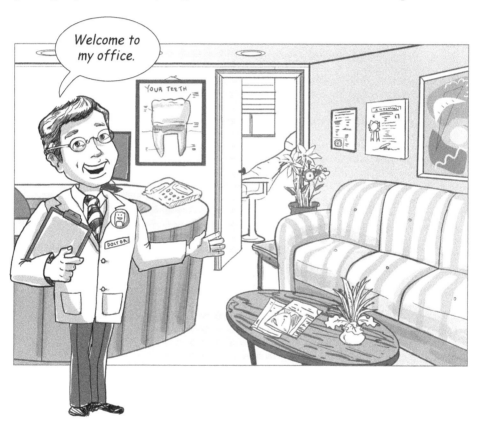

The competition for acceptance into these programs is keen. During their extensive training, periodontists become proficient in the latest techniques and advances in diagnosis and treatment. Following the successful completion of the specialty program, the periodontist receives a postdoctoral certificate. Depending on the country and region, further testing may be required prior to being able to announce oneself as specialist in periodontics (or periodontology), the treatment of periodontal diseases and the placement and maintenance of dental implants.

Taking Your History

Medical History   Using a detailed questionnaire as a guide, the periodontist will ask about your general health. He or she will be interested to know about your diet, smoking history, current medications, allergies and sensitivities to drugs. Recent changes in your general health will be of special importance. If you have a history of heart disease, lung disease, diabetes, nerve disorders, psychological problems or tumors, the periodontist will want to confer with your physician to see how this information could influence the course of your disease and its treatment.

Certain medications, such as oral contraceptives, anti-depressants, and heart medicines, can affect your oral health and the appearance of the gums. It is important to update all your health care providers regarding any medications you are taking, and changes in your general health. Medical conditions can be influenced by periodontal disease, as you will read later on.

Dental History   This part of the discussion usually includes questions such as: When was the patient first told or recognized that gum disease was present? Has there been any treatment? What plaque control methods are in current use? Does the patient understand the importance of daily plaque removal? This last question is pertinent to the successful treatment of periodontal disease. Patients need to be aware that their motivation and participation are key factors. There will also be many questions relating to current and previous dental care. What brought you to the dentist previously? Do you have any special concerns about your mouth, such as esthetics?

Head and Face Exam

After completing the history, attention is given to the exterior of the head, face and neck, looking for any abnormalities in shape or size. This examination is important in revealing swelling, changes in skin texture or coloration, and will include palpation of the glands in the neck.

The TM joint or TMJ (temporomandibular joint) is a part of the jaw located in front of the ear that acts as a hinge (Fig. 5-1). To find the TMJ, place your fingers just in front of the opening to your ear canal; you will feel the movement of these joints as you open and close your jaws. Damage to the TMJ and its associated muscles, which can result from accidents and bite problems, are termed TM disorders. The symptoms of TM disorders include popping, cracking or clicking in the area of the ear, a history of soreness in the jaw, and

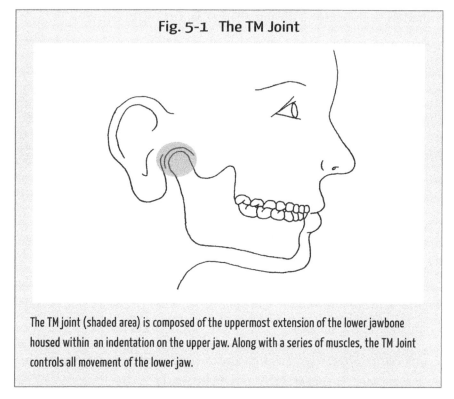

Fig. 5-1 The TM Joint

The TM joint (shaded area) is composed of the uppermost extension of the lower jawbone housed within an indentation on the upper jaw. Along with a series of muscles, the TM Joint controls all movement of the lower jaw.

severe wear of the teeth. It has been noted that patients with TM disorders may also suffer from headaches, dizziness, as well as neck and shoulder pains.

The Periodontal Examination

A detailed look into the mouth is next. Identifying the amount of plaque and calculus that is present is necessary. Gum color, consistency, type, quantity and quality, and level of inflammation will be noted. The periodontist will be interested in knowing if teeth are sensitive during eating, brushing, or as a result of instrument contact. Areas of food impaction, teeth that are rotated or otherwise out of normal position will be recorded. A careful observation will be made of missing teeth, as well as the quality of various dental treatments you have had to date. Old fillings and crowns will be evaluated to determine if they need repair or replacement.

Diagnostic Tests Occasionally the use of one or more tests may be required to assist in establishing a correct diagnosis or in assessing the extent of disease activity. A biopsy requires the removal of a small portion of tissue for microscopic examination. It is essential for evaluating suspicious growths. Blood studies may be indicated if medical problems are suspected of complicating the periodontal condition.

Cultures or other bacteria-identifying examinations can be helpful in developing the precise anti-infective treatment that will be prescribed for you. Sampling of gum fluids found in the sulcus may indicate the level of disease activity.

Genetic profiling, though not widely in use, in the future will likely become a more common technique to identify patients susceptible to advanced gum disease.

Oral Cancer Screening Evaluation of the lips, tongue, floor of the mouth, palate, cheeks and throat will be made to check for any signs of oral cancer. Although oral cancer is fortunately not frequently found, an early diagnosis is critical.

The Periodontal Probe: A Key Investigating Tool

The fundamental tool used in the examination is the periodontal probe. This is a miniature ruler, especially designed to measure the gum sulcus or crevice. On its face are notches at calibrated intervals of one or more millimeters. The probe is placed between the tooth and gum until some resistance is felt, indicating where the gum is attached to the tooth (Fig. 5-2). Normal measurements range up to three millimeters, which translates to a maximum of 1/8 inch (the size of a normal sulcus). In general, any measurement above three millimeters may be considered a periodontal pocket; damage can be

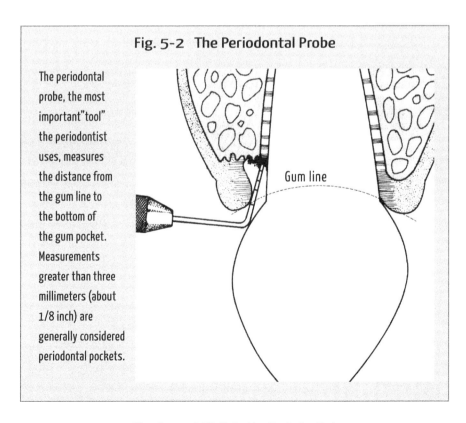

Fig. 5-2 The Periodontal Probe

The periodontal probe, the most important "tool" the periodontist uses, measures the distance from the gum line to the bottom of the gum pocket. Measurements greater than three millimeters (about 1/8 inch) are generally considered periodontal pockets.

Gum line

expected to have already taken place in that area.

For example, a five-millimeter pocket would generally indicate that some of the tooth-supporting bone has been destroyed. Ten millimeters would suggest that perhaps 80-90% of the bone has been lost. The location and amount of bleeding during probing is also recorded.

A complete analysis will include six measurements around each tooth. Remember, gum lines run along the front, sides and back of teeth. Two hundred measurements in one mouth is normal, and will give a detailed typographical profile of the mouth (Fig. 5-3). You need not worry about the number of measurements. You will hardly notice this procedure. Periodontal probe measurements are often called out by the periodontist and recorded by an assistant.

The otherwise mysterious conversation at this point might sound like "… upper right incisor 5…6…9, upper right molar 5…3…9," and so on in succession until all teeth are recorded. With the completion of this part of the examination, we have a detailed map of all your periodontal pockets.

Checking the Bite

The bite or occlusion is best described as the relationship of the teeth to each other in resting, closed and chewing positions. The patient is asked to chew, and slide the upper teeth over the lower teeth. Areas where excess pressure is noted will be recorded for later use. Teeth with abnormal wear or movement will also be noted. Plaster molds of the teeth may be made for further study.

Tooth Movement

Tooth movement or mobility is an important sign of excess tooth pressure and/or periodontal disease. Each tooth is tested. The results are transformed into a number system. Again, working in millimeters, the indications of mobility are "one," two," or "three"

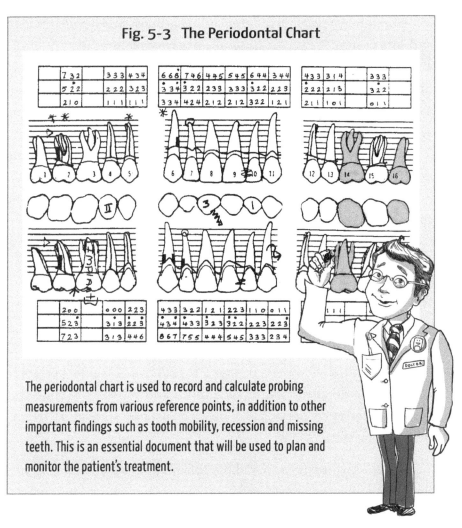

Fig. 5-3 The Periodontal Chart

The periodontal chart is used to record and calculate probing measurements from various reference points, in addition to other important findings such as tooth mobility, recession and missing teeth. This is an essential document that will be used to plan and monitor the patient's treatment.

which signify the degree of movement. "One" is considered early mobility. "Three," which is about 1/8 of an inch side to side, would be very significant movement. Sometimes patients are unaware of mobile teeth.

X-Rays

The examination thus far has involved those areas directly visible to the therapist. The use of x-rays or radiographs provides essential information by revealing differences in hardness and density in hard and soft tissues. X-rays are generally negative pictures in gray, black, and white. The whiter the image the greater the density. A silver filling or gold cap would appear white because radiation does not easily pass through. The tongue, gums and cheeks appear dark and are not readily discernible.

Radiographs allow the detection of early bone breakdown around teeth as well as the size and shape of roots, cavities, cysts, signs of bite trauma, the need for a possible root canal, extra teeth and bone tumors. There are three major types of x-rays used in dentistry.

Panoramic   One is the panoramic x-ray in which a general view of all the teeth and jaws is shown in a single large rectangular view.

Full Mouth Series   A second type, which is preferred in the diagnosis of periodontal disease, is a complete set of periapical x-rays (also known as full mouth series) taken of individual teeth or groups of teeth. When the views are arranged together in a frame, periapical x-rays give a detailed view of each tooth and supporting bone. The complete series of periapical x-rays consists of sixteen to twenty individual views.

CT Scan   A third type of radiograph may be suggested if dental implants are being considered, or if there is need for more precise details of a suspicious area. A CT scan (computerized tomography) reveals specific areas of the jaw in three dimensions. These x-rays can then be studied by your surgeon to determine the best surgical approach.

Periodontal Disease and Medical Conditions

The relationship between periodontal disease and medical conditions or diseases has generated both great interest and concern. There is increasing evidence suggesting that the presence of advanced

Fig. 5-4 X-Rays

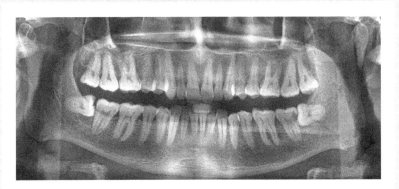

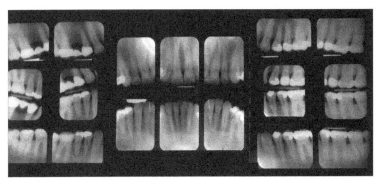

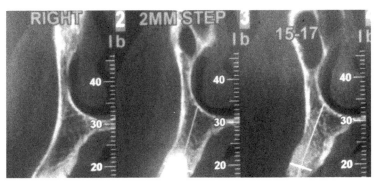

The panoramic x-ray (above) gives a general view of the mouth and jaws, while the full mouth series (center) shows details of each tooth and its surrounding area. The CT (below) provides detailed 3-d views of the mouth allowing the therapist to view highly detailed longitudinal "slices" of the area in question- most often used for implant treatment planning.

periodontal disease may influence the initiation and/or the course of certain medical problems. The reader is cautioned however, that further research is needed before an irrefutable cause and effect relationship can be established for most of the suggested or reported relationships.

One popular hypothesis suggests that the gum disease-causing bacteria, its toxins and/or the accumulation of responding elements in the body's defensive system extend their influence beyond the mouth, allowing areas far removed from your teeth to become endangered.

There is considerable controversy on many of the purported associations between gum disease and systemic health, though all those mentioned in this chapter have been discussed in respected professional journals and at prestigious scientific meetings. Most of the public however, have received their information from the media, which has attracted much attention to the subject with provocative and often misleading headlines such as "Floss or Die". Briefly listed below are some of the most frequently reported gum disease-systemic relationships; however, for a more in-depth understanding of the impact of a periodontal disease on your systemic health, consult with your dentist or periodontist.

Diabetes

Diabetic patients are more likely to develop periodontal disease, which in turn can increase blood sugar and diabetic complications.

People with diabetes, especially those whose diabetes are poorly controlled, are more likely to have serious gum disease than those without diabetes. Today, periodontal disease is considered by many endocrinologists (specialists in the treatment of diabetes) to be a complication of diabetes.

Research has for many years suggested that the relationship between diabetes and periodontal disease is such that not only can diabetes exacerbate an already existing periodontal disease, but also untreated periodontal infections can affect the patient's ability to control insulin levels.

Heart/ Cardiovascular Diseases

Several studies have shown an association between periodontal disease and heart disease. While a cause-and-effect relationship has not yet been proven, research has indicated that periodontal disease increases the risk of heart disease. Scientists believe that inflammation caused by periodontal disease may be responsible for the association.

Periodontal disease can also exacerbate existing heart conditions. Patients at risk for infective endocarditis (an infection on the valves of your heart) may require antibiotics prior to dental procedures.

Your periodontist and cardiologist will be able to determine if your heart condition requires use of antibiotics prior to dental procedures. Studies have also suggested a relationship between periodontal disease and stroke. In one particular study, oral infection was seen as a risk factor for stroke in people diagnosed with acute heart disease.

Osteoporosis

Research is pointing to the possibility that osteoporosis leads to tooth loss because the quality of the tooth-supporting bone has deteriorated.

Respiratory Disease

Periodontal disease causing bacteria can travel from the mouth into the lungs, contributing to the development of serious diseases such as pneumonia.

Cancer

A study published in the highly respected journal *The Lancet Oncology* and widely reported, including by the American Academy of Periodontology, 48,000 men were asked about their periodontal disease experience and other diseases.

Researchers found that men with gum disease were 49% more likely to develop kidney cancer, 54% more likely to develop pancreatic cancer, and 30% more likely to develop blood cancers. While the results are disturbing, it is important to remember that these conclusions still require further study, and at this point only make the suggestion that there is an association between gum disease and cancer, but do not prove a cause-and-effect relationship. Much more study is required.

Prostate Health

Usually found only in small amounts, the levels of Prostate-specific antigen, PSA, increases when the prostate is inflamed, infected, or cancerous. Men with signs of gum inflammation demonstrate a higher PSA than those with only one of the conditions. This suggests that prostate health may influence or be connected with periodontal health.

Impotence

Men younger than 30 or older than 70, are more likely to report impotence. Research has suggested that inflammation may be the culprit; prolonged chronic inflammation, like periodontal disease, can damage blood vessels leading to impotence.

And There's More

In addition to the above, the following diseases or conditions have also been implicated as having a relationship with periodontal disease and have been reported in peer-reviewed, scientific journals: chronic obstructive pulmonary disease, chronic kidney disease, rheumatoid arthritis, cognitive impairment, obesity, metabolic syndrome and preterm, low birth weight pregnancy outcomes.

6

The Prognosis

Forcasting the Future of Your Teeth

How Long Will I Keep My Teeth?

After completing the evaluation process, the periodontist will meet with the patient to review the information obtained during the examination, the results of any laboratory tests and the x-ray findings. In addition, the patient will be presented with a suggested plan of treatment (more on this in the next chapter), the time involved and the expected fee.

There will be a discussion about the specific nature of his/her periodontal disease. Educational materials will be offered on the subject, which not only explain the disease, but go a long way in reassuring the patient that he or she is not alone. In fact, many people are comforted to know that they do not have a rare disease.

Once patients understand their periodontal disease and the proposed treatment, it is not uncommon to hear the question "Okay, if I complete the treatment, pay the fee and follow directions, how long will I keep my teeth?"

Prognosis is the technique of forecasting the future of your teeth, based on the anticipated course of the disease in conjunction with the opportunity to provide appropriate treatment. Just as the meteorologist relies on many sources of data to forecast the weather,

Ignore Your Teeth and They'll Go Away

so periodontists need to harness all their accumulated scientific skills and experience to establish an accurate and reliable forecast or prognosis of the teeth.

Risk Factors No two patients are exactly alike. Some may appear similar at first, but will yield quite different results. This is because periodontal disease is a multi-factorial disease. In other words, although we know that plaque is the primary cause of gum disease, there are other influences that modify the character of the disease and the determination of the prognosis. Sometimes these influences are referred to as risk factors, because they may place patients at risk for more serious periodontal problems.

The various risk factors that influence the disease process and prognosis are identified prior to the start of therapy to assist in establishing a treatment plan suited to the individual patient. For purposes of clarity, these factors have been divided into two areas. General risk factors affect the individual as a whole and could also impact on other health problems or conditions. Many of these factors help determine the patient's host response as discussed in Chapter 3. Local risk factors tend to have a more direct effect on the oral structures.

General Risk Factors

Systemic Diseases

Systemic diseases and/or the medications associated with their treatment may increase the severity of periodontal disease. The more common examples include those that interfere with the body's ability to fight infections, such as rheumatoid arthritis, diabetes, compromised immunity conditions, blood diseases and cardiovascular illnesses.

Stress

There are suggestive scientific findings, which indicate that stress can have a significant effect on the severity of gum disease, as well as an adverse influence on the body's response to treatment.

Genetics

We now have the ability to locate specific genetic factors that predict susceptibility to gum disease. Although not in widespread use, the potential application of this information has created great promise for identifying patients who are at particular risk for advanced periodontal disease.

Smoking

Smokers are more likely to build up excessive calculus, unsightly stains and bad breath. Research has confirmed that tobacco use leads to gum recession, mouth sores, deeper periodontal pockets and a greater chance of loosing one's teeth. The results of therapy will also be compromised. It should be noted that smokeless tobacco has similar effects as smoking on periodontal health and both types of tobacco use increase significantly the risk of oral cancer.

Age

Surprisingly, for two patients with the same amount of disease, the prognosis is better for the older patient than for the younger one. The reason is that the older individual has managed to preserve a certain amount of bone for a long period of time. Losing bone slowly, while undesirable, is still the expected course for untreated periodontal disease. The younger patient, having a rapid-type bone loss, suggests that additional influences need to be addressed (see aggressive periodontitis in Chapter 3).

Special Problems for Women

Changes in women's hormonal balance may influence the reaction of gum tissue to plaque and calculus. Women are particularly susceptible to gum problems during puberty, menstruation, pregnancy, menopause and while taking oral contraceptives.

For example, a pregnancy tumor, while not a true tumor, describes a localized growth of gum tissue usually found between the teeth, often seen during pregnancy. This growth, known as pyogenic granuloma, is due to a heightened response of the gum tissue to irritation. Also, osteoporosis, a common problem after the age of 50, can weaken tooth-supporting bone. In addition, the medications that are used to treat osteoporosis can negatively impact the healing of bone following periodontal and implant surgery.

Poor Nutrition and Obesity

Improper diet may influence periodontal health. Usually it takes a severe vitamin deficiency to affect a noticeable gum change. However, all the body systems and organs are influenced by the proper intake of a nutritious and balanced diet. A poor diet may alter the ability of the gum tissue to resist infection, as well as respond effectively to treatment. A number of studies have shown that obesity may also be a risk factor.

Local Risk Factors

Plaque Control

The patient's ability to maintain low levels of plaque and the motivation to continue doing so after active treatment, are fundamental to the success of therapy and insuring a better prognosis.

Something About Melanie

Melanie is a young woman who appeared for her regular examination complaining about bleeding gums. Melanie always demonstrated excellent oral hygiene and very little buildup of plaque or tartar. But that day, even though there wasn't much plaque, there was quite a bit of bleeding. So I asked her; "By any chance Melanie are you pregnant?" She told me, with tears swelling up in her eyes, that she and her husband had been trying to have a baby for several years, and being unsuccessful, had given up and were planning to adopt. They were traveling the next week to a foreign country to start a complicated and expensive adoption procedure. I suggested that she go to her physician and get a blood test.

Melanie had plenty of disappointments in the past few years, but agreed to my suggestion. Needless to say, her blood test was positive for pregnancy. Eight months later, Melanie and Jim had a beautiful baby boy. The inflammation and bleeding caused by the excess in hormones was controlled with frequent hygiene visits throughout the entire term of her pregnancy. I guess you could say this was one of those times when bad news (gum inflammation) was really good news!

From my files...

Ignore Your Teeth and They'll Go Away

Pocket Depth

Numerous studies have shown that the deeper the pocket the more difficult it is to treat and the more likely that there will be disease progression. Therefore, teeth with shallower pockets will generally have a better prognosis.

Amount of Supporting Bone

The amount of remaining bone, which supports the tooth, is crucial. If bone loss is extensive the prognosis is negatively affected.

Number of Remaining Teeth

If the number and distribution of remaining teeth are inadequate to support replacements, such as bridges or removable partials, the prognosis is likely to be poor. The weakened teeth will be compromised by having to absorb excess biting pressures.

Loose Teeth

Teeth that show increasing looseness due to periodontal disease are more likely to suffer additional bone loss and disease progression.

Tooth Root Anatomy

A long root has a greater amount of supporting bone. The loss of, let's say, a 1/4 of an inch of bone on a long root would not be as harmful as the same amount of bone loss around a short root. Molar teeth have more than one root (Fig. 6-1). Furcation involvement, an infection that invades the bone between the roots, creates special problems for treatment and a definite poorer prognosis.

Bad Bite

A bad bite is known as malocclusion, and occurs when the teeth do

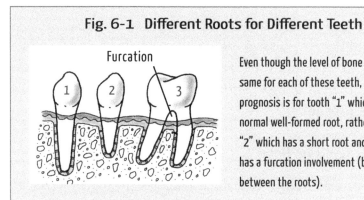

Fig. 6-1 Different Roots for Different Teeth

Furcation

Even though the level of bone loss is the same for each of these teeth, the best prognosis is for tooth "1" which has a normal well-formed root, rather than for "2" which has a short root and "3" which has a furcation involvement (bone loss between the roots).

not meet properly when you bite or chew your food. Because the bite is actually uneven, some teeth may absorb greater stress than they were designed for, and shift or loosen within their bone sockets. The longer this continues, the more the teeth become weaker and sensitive. Crowded, rotated and loose teeth are also susceptible targets for plaque build-up, leading to gum disease.

Tooth Grinding

Clenching or grinding one's teeth is called bruxism. Many people suffer from this habit unknowingly in their sleep. During bruxism, excessive pressures are generated by the jaw musculature on the teeth. If this process occurs on teeth already suffering from periodontal disease, the bone loss can be accelerated (see Chapter 5, Head and Face Exam).

Poor Dental Work

Weakened, cracked or ill-fitting fillings and crowns lead to the accumulation of plaque, which promotes gum disease (Fig. 6-2). Loose partial dentures and unstable connections to the teeth can weaken the supporting teeth and irritate gum tissues.

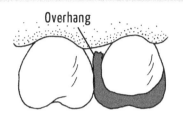

Fig. 6-2 Filling Overhang

Overhang

In this illustration, an overhang, a poorly shaped filling or restoration is demonstrated, which can contribute to plaque accumulation and gum disease.

Influence of the Therapist

In addition to the local and general factors, an important influence on the overall response to treatment must include the therapist's skill and experience. Needless to say, as the disease progresses or becomes more complicated, advanced treatment is required. Selecting a therapist whose skill and experience includes an expertise in the full range of periodontal treatments and diagnoses will enhance the prognosis.

Range of Prognosis

An analysis is made of all the accumulated information, including the local and general risk factors. A prediction is then made of the future of your teeth. The range of prognosis may include the following terms: Good, Fair, Guarded and Hopeless.

Good   indicates that there is strong reason to believe that the teeth will respond to periodontal therapy and may not even need advanced treatment in order to be maintained for life.

Fair indicates that the chances of success are realistic. Some bone loss has occurred; surgical therapy may be required. However, with appropriate follow-up treatment the teeth could be expected to last for many years.

Guarded (also "poor" or "questionable") would signify that even if treatment is rendered, the chances for complete success are limited. Teeth that are saved may need to be joined together for mutual support.

Hopeless means there is no reasonable possibility of being able to save the tooth; the disease is too advanced, and the damage too severe. These teeth usually need to be removed.

The most detailed prognosis includes a prediction for each tooth as well as all the teeth together as one functioning unit.

The prognosis clearly spells out the course the disease is likely to take, as well as the chances for the successful treatment and maintenance of the teeth. One should keep in mind that during and after treatment, the prognosis might change (for better or worse) as a result of the patient's response to therapy.

With the prognosis established, the patient is ready to begin the treatment phase.

PART III
Treatment

7

Plaque Control

Everyday Care for
Your Teeth and Gums

The First Step

Recalling that the chief cause of gum disease is bacterial plaque, it is logical that treatment is directed towards eliminating this primary cause.

Unless there is an emergency, the first step in the treatment of gum disease is adopting an effective oral disease control program aimed at achieving as plaque-free a mouth as possible. Every dental professional will approach this challenge in a different way, including the use of demonstration videos and booklets to help patients understand their disease.

It's in your hands.

This is the most important topic of the book, because it deals with what you can do to help arrest your disease and save your teeth; and for those without gum disease, following the advice in this chapter can go along way towards preventing you from developing serious gum problems. Please read it carefully.

Controlling Plaque Every Day

The single most important treatment anyone can do for gum disease is daily plaque removal using scientifically proven techniques.

You will probably need to change the way you clean your teeth. Old habits will have to be abandoned. New methods will be a bother, a time-consuming nuisance, until you establish new patterns. But nothing else will solve your problem. No pill has yet been developed, which rids plaque from your mouth!

Look at it this way: if your present cleaning ritual was doing the job, you would have no need for periodontal treatment. So, recognizing that you need to change your methods is a good start.

You can not clean your teeth too often. Many therapists recommend cleaning after every meal. This is perhaps an idealistic goal that few can actually achieve. Experts would agree that one thorough cleaning a day is preferable to three or more cursory ones.

How do you brush your teeth now? Up and down? Or with a horizontal scrubbing motion that is easier and more natural? Do you use a hard brush or soft? Natural bristles or nylon? Toothpaste, gel or powder? Floss or toothpicks?

As a result of scientific studies, many of the long accepted ideas about tooth brushing have been discarded. And yet there are still many variations of accepted brushing techniques. This is because each patient's teeth are different and have unique problems with plaque control. Your therapist will give you specific instructions on the best methods for cleaning your teeth.

Disclosing Plaque   To effectively remove plaque you need to see it. For this purpose, a disclosing solution or tablet (available at most pharmacies) may be used containing a dye that stains and identifies plaque. Patients are instructed how to apply the dye. Observing your teeth at this time will reveal areas of plaque accumulation where oral hygiene procedures need to be improved.

Brushing

Proper brushing techniques ensure that all accessible surfaces of each tooth and the tongue are thoroughly cleaned.

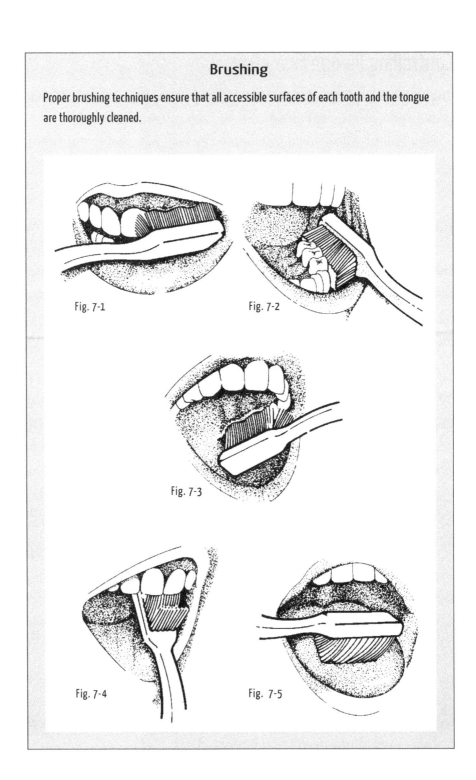

Fig. 7-1

Fig. 7-2

Fig. 7-3

Fig. 7-4

Fig. 7-5

Tooth Brushing

First, use the toothbrush dry and with no toothpaste. Starting on the outside upper or lower molars, hold the brush parallel to the gum line and at a 45° angle to the tooth (Fig.7-1). Applying enough pressure so that the bristles can get into the sulcus between gum and tooth, brush with five or six very short strokes, just enough to move the bristles back and forth on two or three teeth at a time. It should be a vibrating motion aimed at cleaning just the area that can be covered by the bristles at one time.

After several short strokes, turn the handle of the brush in your hand so that the bristles sweep from the gum toward the top of the teeth. Then move the brush around the mouth and repeat the procedure until you have cleaned the outer side of all the teeth, top and bottom (Fig. 7-2).

Now, begin the same process on the inner side (Fig. 7-3). You will find that it is easy to jiggle the brush and sweep away from the gum on the sides. It may be more difficult to brush in the same way behind your front teeth (Fig. 7-4). For this area a smaller brush may be recommended. Don't forget to brush your tongue. Many bacteria settle within the crevices of this large muscle (Fig. 7-5). Note that toothpaste is not used during this step.

Flossing

Most serious gum disease occurs between the teeth where brushing cannot reach. This is why so many patients who brush religiously are shocked to discover that they are in jeopardy of losing their teeth. If the space between the teeth is not cleaned, gum disease may occur.

Floss is our chief weapon for this area. Many people think dental floss is only for dislodging bits of food trapped between their teeth. To prevent gum disease however, flossing should be done as often as brushing or at least once a day.

Flossing

Flossing, though technically more difficult than brushing, is required to reach the areas between the teeth that the toothbrush cannot reach.

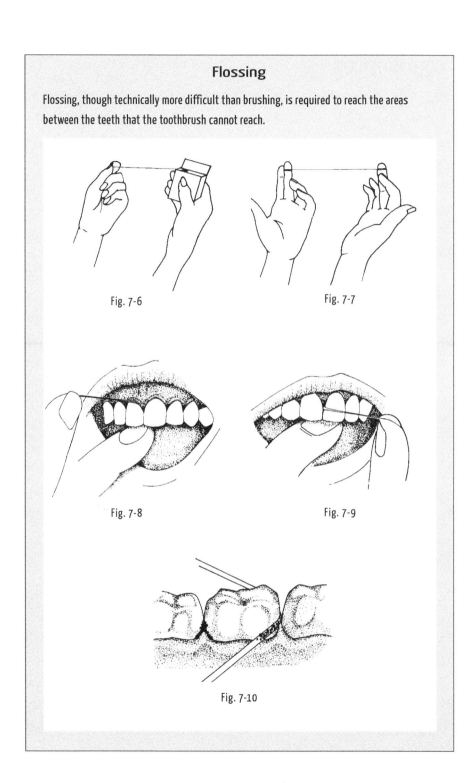

Fig. 7-6

Fig. 7-7

Fig. 7-8

Fig. 7-9

Fig. 7-10

If you do it correctly, you will use one to two feet of dental floss each time. If that seems like a lot, consider that it is just one or two inches of floss per tooth. The best approach is to hold the dental floss dispenser in one hand. Pull out about eighteen inches of floss (Fig. 7-6) and take one turn around the middle finger on the hand holding the dispenser. Now anchor the end of the floss by taking two or three turns around the middle finger of the other hand, leaving five or six inches of floss between the two hands (Fig. 7-7).

Then, using both index fingers to guide the floss, place it around the sides of one of your front teeth. Bring the floss gently down into the sulcus between tooth and gum and pull the ends of the floss forward to form a tight "C" around the base of the tooth, (Fig. 7-8) then lift the floss up along the side of the tooth toward the top and slide over to the adjacent tooth (Fig. 7-9). Floss that breaks or sheds may indicate the need to replace weak fillings or crowns.

As you finish one tooth, allow another short length of floss to pull out of the dispenser and take up the slack by taking another wrap around your middle finger. This technique provides a clean length of floss for each tooth and prevents carrying plaque from one pocket to another.

In slipping the floss between the teeth, be careful not to pull so hard that the floss is jerked into the gum. These tissues are tender and can be injured if the floss is handled roughly. You will soon develop a routine for flossing both sides of each tooth in turn. It is not important where you start or finish. The main thing is to be sure that you remove the plaque as completely as possible from both sides of each tooth (Fig. 7-10).

Toothpaste

When flossing is finished, you are ready for toothpaste and a final brushing. Toothpaste is useful as a breath freshener and tooth polish, but it is relatively ineffective in removing plaque. This is why

A Brushing Lesson for Jeremy's Parents

I often go to local elementary and nursery schools to teach children basic tooth brushing and proper nutrition. So when my good patients Brad and Mary asked me to visit little Jeremy's 1st grade health day, I was happy to oblige. It's also a non-threatening environment in which to make a good first impression about dentistry on young children.

I was amazed however that these very conscientious parents actually asked me why it was necessary to brush their children's baby teeth since they'll be falling out anyway. In my experience, many parents have expressed similar misunderstandings. So I explained to Brad and Mary that the first point I raise with the children, during my visits, is how important their first set of teeth are and why taking good care of them is not an option, but a necessity! I emphasize this by reminding them and their teachers, "don't forget to tell your parents and make sure they get a copy of the hygiene instructions." Effective dental cleaning habits should start when the first tooth appears in the mouth by gently holding the child and rubbing a cotton pellet or soft cloth along the teeth. It should feel comfortable. As children grow older, they can start to brush by themselves with the supervision of their parents.

From my files...

you need to do the plaque control steps first. Some toothpastes have additives that assist in retarding the accumulation of plaque and tartar, fluoride to reduce decay and other ingredients that can help control gingivitis.

Again, the recommended technique is to brush away from the gums toward the top of the tooth so that the bristles can sweep into the spaces between the gum and tooth. Most toothpastes are acceptable, but your therapist may recommend a special toothpaste depending on your individual dental condition.

For Improved Plaque Control

For Tight Spaces Patients with fixed bridges or very tight spaces may find normal flossing impossible. In these areas, specially designed loops are used which thread the floss into the spaces between the teeth and/or under the bridge. Floss holders act like fingers making it easier to reach difficult areas with the floss. Narrow brushes that fit between the teeth are often recommended for patients as a substitute or in addition to flossing when adequate space exists to accommodate the brush.

Aids, which stimulate the gum tissues such as rubber tips and wood sticks, may be used to help firm the gum tissues through a massaging effect, and to assist in the removal of retained food particles and plaque.

Electric Toothbrushes are effective for the removal of food debris and plaque. An electric toothbrush can be helpful for the handicapped as well as for those who otherwise find it difficult to manipulate manual brushes. Some patients enjoy the novelty of the electric toothbrush, which may encourage better brushing habits. It is important to realize that regardless of the brushing technique, the plaque must be removed in order to be effective. So if you find a particular type of brush that makes cleaning your teeth easier and more comfortable, that's the one to choose.

Mouth Rinses and Oral Irrigation   Mouth rinses and other chemical solutions are often advertised as preventing bad breath. Some solutions have been shown to be effective in controlling plaque and improving gingivitis. An oral irrigator which permits the solutions to be delivered directly and efficiently into the periodontal pocket may be recommended after the patient receives instructions by the therapist. Chlorhexidine is one of the most widely prescribed chemical agents of this type.

Periodontists will often recommend these agents as a supplement to other therapies, when additional support for plaque control is required. The patient is instructed regarding the correct method and the period of time that these solutions are to be used. As some of the solutions are potent antimicrobial agents, it is important to follow the directions carefully, and not to undertake or change the regimen without professional consultation.

Diet and Periodontal Disease

In general, a balanced diet will help to assure that your vital organs and other body systems are working at maximum efficiency. While

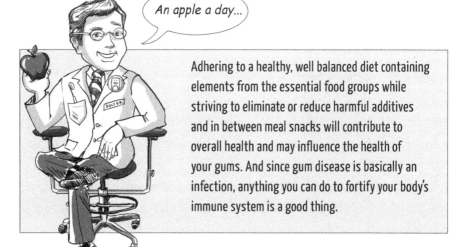

An apple a day...

Adhering to a healthy, well balanced diet containing elements from the essential food groups while striving to eliminate or reduce harmful additives and in between meal snacks will contribute to overall health and may influence the health of your gums. And since gum disease is basically an infection, anything you can do to fortify your body's immune system is a good thing.

Ignore Your Teeth and They'll Go Away

there is little evidence of a direct correlation between general nutrition and periodontal disease, it is reasonable to assume that when a patient's general health suffers from the lack of a healthy diet, the body's ability to fight off gum infection may be impaired. A poor diet can also influence the quality of recovery following surgical procedures. As noted previously, obesity can contribute to increase risk for periodontal disease.

Of course, sugar specifically has a direct effect on the mouth. Not only is it responsible for dental decay, but the crevices created by decay can also contribute to plaque retention. The reader is referred to the many excellent guides to nutrition for establishing a balanced healthy diet.

One Day at a Time

If all these changes in the care of your mouth seem like a heavy burden, perhaps it is best not to think too far in the future. Try taking one day at a time. Start with one aid and one area of the mouth and work your way up to a comprehensive routine. To check your overall brushing and flossing efficiency, try to use plaque-disclosing material once every other day after oral hygiene procedures for the first two weeks, followed by once a week as a continual check.

With most periodontal diseases, you are really much more fortunate than patients suffering from the majority of medical ailments. Few can actually take direct action, which will arrest or reverse their disease.

With the help of your periodontist or family dentist to advise and provide treatment as necessary, the patient who develops an effective program of plaque control can cure early gum disease and better maintain the results of treatment.

8

Initial Therapy

Primary Treatment for Most Periodontal Diseases

First Treatment Phase

While the patient is learning to effectively remove plaque, a series of treatments is usually performed, aimed at reducing the causes and influences within the mouth which are responsible for periodontal disease. These procedures, which include plaque control, are non-surgical, generally the first phase of actual treatment, and are often collectively termed initial therapy.

Scaling

In combination with plaque control, removing local irritants and preventing their recurrence, improve nearly all forms of gum disease. The process of removing plaque and tartar from the teeth is known as scaling. Your dentist may have scaled your teeth as part of a procedure commonly known as cleaning. A cleaning however may not include scaling, especially in the case of patients without gum disease, and is often limited to a cursory removal of stain.

Root Planing

Technically, scaling only removes the calculus and other substances

Ignore Your Teeth and They'll Go Away

on the tooth's surfaces. The upper portion of the tooth or crown is covered by hard enamel, while the root is covered by a softer substance known as cementum, which can easily be damaged, or contaminated by retained calculus, plaque and bacteria. Root planing is a delicate smoothing of the rough or irregular root surface to enhance the reattachment of gum tissue and retard additional plaque formation. Historically, this procedure was done more aggressively as it can lead to increased sensitivity and root exposure. Today therapists are careful to retain as much cementum as possible while performing this procedure. In fact, many specialists do not utilize root planing as a separate procedure independent of scaling.

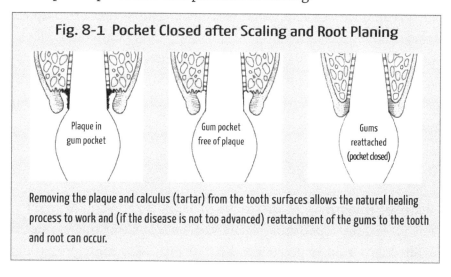

Fig. 8-1 Pocket Closed after Scaling and Root Planing

Plaque in gum pocket

Gum pocket free of plaque

Gums reattached (pocket closed)

Removing the plaque and calculus (tartar) from the tooth surfaces allows the natural healing process to work and (if the disease is not too advanced) reattachment of the gums to the tooth and root can occur.

For Your Comfort

During scaling and root planing you may receive a local anesthetic injection or anesthetic paste to eliminate discomfort. Scaling and root planing utilize a variety of specialized instruments to remove plaque and tartar. This wide range of options makes it possible to comfortably gain access to deposits above and below the gum line. Most of the time, these procedures do not cause pain. However, some patients are nevertheless more relaxed with the area anesthetized.

You may be scheduled from one to six or more appointments to complete scaling and root planing which may be performed in segments. The segments are usually made up of quarters of the mouth known as quadrants (up to eight teeth). Your therapist may treat one or two quadrants at a time. Occasionally the entire mouth can be completed in one session.

The Dental Hygienist

Dental hygienists are essential, trained, professional members of the periodontal therapy team, and may (under the direction of the periodontist or family dentist) undertake partial or complete responsibility for scaling, root planing, motivation and plaque control. The dental hygienist is also trained to perform a wide variety of additional duties including periodontal probing, taking of impressions for diagnostic models, x-rays and application of various medications.

Polishing

The final smoothing of the tooth surfaces is called polishing. For this procedure, a polishing agent such as a paste of fine pumice is applied to a rubber polishing cup or brush. Any remaining tooth discoloration may be removed as well. Fluoride may be applied after polishing, because of its ability to reduce sensitivity and its known anti-decay properties.

Correcting Worn or Poor Fitting Dental Work

You may have discovered difficulty flossing in areas where old fillings or poor fitting crowns were found (see Fig. 6-2). These problems can limit the good results following scaling and root planing, and

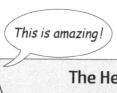

This is amazing!

The Healing Process in Your Mouth

More than anything else, successful treatment of early gum disease is predictable because of the remarkable capacity of the gum tissues to heal and repair following the removal of plaque and tartar, and improvement in oral hygiene (see Fig. 8-1).

Think of an embedded wood splinter that separates two sides of skin. The splinter is acting as an irritant. As long as it remains the skin will not join back together. And yet, soon after the splinter is removed, the skin begins to repair itself until the separation disappears. This is similar to what happens after scaling and root planing.

Following removal of the irritants, which are the plaque and calculus (represented by the splinter analogy), the gum pocket fills with a microscopic blood clot which will convert to healthy tissues. Within a day or two, the inner gum lining begins to heal, and is often reattached to the tooth by the end of two weeks. Usually, if the disease is caught early enough, consistency, contour and texture of the gums will return to health, and the gum margin will adapt to the tooth.

contribute to further retention of plaque. Therefore, the correction of these obstacles to effective oral hygiene will, when possible, be accomplished as part of the initial procedures by your dentist in consultation with the periodontist. In addition, removal of active decay, required root canal therapy or extraction of hopeless teeth may also be completed at this time.

Treating Bite Problems

Irregularity in the bite or malocclusion is an important consideration in the treatment of periodontal disease. When the teeth do not meet evenly or are positioned improperly in the mouth, gum disease can be exacerbated.

Occlusal (Bite) Adjustment   Occlusal adjustment involves the reshaping or smoothing of the tooth's biting surfaces so the bite becomes gradually more even and the pressures balanced throughout the mouth.

For this procedure a hand-piece or rotary drill is utilized that allows a minimal amount of tooth material to be removed or reshaped.

The patient is asked to bring the teeth together during normal chewing strokes. A strip of inked, thin paper is held between the teeth. When the paper is removed, pressure points are seen where the teeth came together. The darker pressure points represent areas that need reshaping.

Occlusal adjustment is not painful. This treatment may involve one or more appointments depending on the severity of the problem. Most patients find that following occlusal adjustment their bite is more comfortable and their teeth have an improved sense of "belonging together."

Bite Guard Therapy   Patients with a grinding or clenching habit, called bruxism, exert excessive stress on the teeth. To alleviate these problems, a bite guard is made (Fig. 8-2). This removable appliance is designed from models taken of the patient's teeth. Bite guards are usually made of a hard plastic that fit over the upper or lower teeth. The bite guard is designed to be worn during periods of bruxism. For many, this is during sleep. Others find it necessary at work or when they pursue concentrated tasks. For some (especially those in acute pain), the wearing of a bite guard may be required twenty-four hours a day.

Use of the bite guard may eliminate the habit of bruxism, however most patients continue to grind or clench and must wear the bite guard for an extended period of time. Patients often report relief from the symptoms of TM Disorders (discussed on the following page) after wearing the bite guard. The appliance must be checked for evidence of wear. Adjustments are often required.

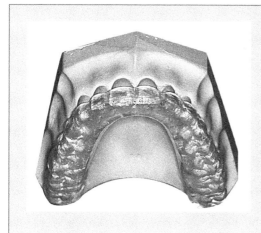

Fig. 8-2 Bite Guard

A bite guard is made usually from a clear plastic material and fitted to the upper teeth. It may be worn at night or during the day depending on when the patient is grinding his or her teeth. In this photograph, the bite guard is resting on the stone model of the patient's upper teeth.

Orthodontics Orthodontics (straightening of the teeth) may be included during comprehensive periodontal treatment to correct abnormalities that contribute to gum disease or for purely esthetic reasons. Adults are usually surprised to find that with modern orthodontic techniques much of the stigma associated with "braces" has been eliminated. Minor tooth movement is the realignment of teeth that do not require complex techniques. More involved treatment requiring the banding of all teeth, or major realignment of the teeth and jaws may be referred to an orthodontist.

If a patient is considering orthodontics, active gum disease must be eliminated prior to the start of treatment. The braces, brackets and wires used in orthodontics attract plaque and can result in over-growth or infection of the gum tissue. Tooth movement in an infected area can lead to abscesses, rapid destruction of bone and the loss of teeth.

Jerry: It's Not in Your Head

Jerry, a 50-year-old successful businessman and avid health enthusiast, took very good care of his body and with exercise and by eating a healthy balanced diet. He could be found on the high school track running at least three times a week. His only major complaint was the pain and stiffness in his jaws especially after waking up in the morning. I informed Jerry that he had TMJ problems, which meant he was grinding his teeth at night (subconsciously) causing stress not only on his teeth, which were beginning to wear down, but also on the powerful jaw muscles that control the movements of the jaw and the joint found just in the front of the ear called the TMJ (see Fig. 5-1). Jerry also reported that he would frequently wake up with headaches, which required medication several times a week and really put him out of sorts.

Within a few days after having a bite guard placed in his mouth, he began to feel better and soon found himself waking up in the morning refreshed from a good night's sleep without the pain and joint problems. And Jerry's headaches have disappeared.

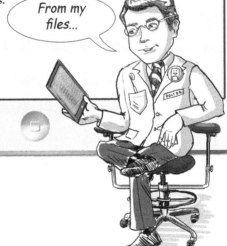

From my files...

Ignore Your Teeth and They'll Go Away

Patients with treated gum disease need to be seen frequently for periodontal monitoring during orthodontic care.

Reevaluation

Usually a waiting period of a few weeks to several months passes before a reevaluation is made regarding further treatment. During reevaluation, many factors are considered. If, for example, periodontal pockets have been reduced, bleeding eliminated and the patient is able to thoroughly remove plaque on a daily basis, no further treatment may be required.

On the other hand, patients with continuing problems such as deep periodontal pockets, continued signs of inflammation, loose teeth and esthetic defects, will benefit from the periodontal surgery discussed in the next chapter.

9

Periodontal Surgery

Options and Alternatives

Considering Gum Surgery

In advanced gum disease, surgery offers the best chance for saving teeth. Periodontal surgery includes a wide variety of techniques and procedures ranging from simply removing gum tissue to the most advanced bone and soft tissue grafting procedures. Various studies have shown that the vast majority of patients who have had periodontal surgery are able to retain most, if not all, of their teeth. This is a reassuring statement. In some cases, weak teeth may eventually be lost. But corrective surgery and follow-up treatment can be given credit for saving the rest. As a patient, your chances of living out your whole life with your own teeth are excellent.

Relax – Reducing Stress Before and After Surgery

Despite having full confidence in their periodontist, and after all the explanations of the true nature of the advanced procedures, it is natural for some patients to still feel apprehensive prior to surgery. Reducing pre-surgery stress enables the body to relax. Allocating time away from a demanding work schedule before surgery for sports or hobbies is a good stress reducer. Remember, stress may be a contributing factor to certain types of gum disease. It may even be

OK, I know surgery sounds serious, but...

A Word (or Two) about the "Word"

To begin with, there is clearly something about the word "surgery" that can have an unsettling effect. That is understandable. Surgery conjures up a sense of serious business. There are, of course, certain risks involved in any procedure, be it a heart transplant or a wart removal. Also, there is no getting away from the fact that any surgical procedure is unpleasant. Its aftermath almost always involves some temporary, although often surprisingly mild, discomfort. The degree of discomfort will vary with each patient.

Apart from the fear of pain, there are the psychological factors stimulated by the announcement that the next step is surgery. Such announcement proclaims to the patient that there is something irrevocably wrong. One can no longer think, "I'm really O.K. I just ought to remember to brush my teeth more often." The recommendation of surgery can be an attack on the patient's basic self-image and triggers complex and unconscious reactions.

One may think it an indictment of the patient's ability to take proper care of one's self. It may be a grim reminder of advancing age and eventual mortality. It recalls the admonition of parents or teachers. It can awaken buried hostilities. It often suggests a measure of personal failure. All these reactions and others affect the patient's response to the need for surgery.

While most patients react with some degree of apprehension when surgery is discussed, many have found that the anticipatory fear far outweighed the reality of the actual experience. Unfortunately, some people who are so paralyzed by the sound of the word surgery, would rather chance having false teeth than undergo the procedure. The tragedy is that these are the individuals who, because they chose not to have surgery, will likely suffer the discomfort, expense and eventual tooth loss they had hoped to avoid.

a significant deterrent to speedy healing. Therefore, managing your tensions may be as important as the actual operating techniques.

Though performing surgery in a very localized area, the conscientious surgeon remembers that the mouth is only a part of the total human being. Therefore, to help the patient relax prior to surgery, the following additional suggestions may be considered.

Medications For patients apprehensive about surgery, tranquilizers or sedatives can be prescribed. Some are taken the night before; others are taken or injected while resting in the office prior to or during the procedure. These medications will calm your fears and allow you to be more relaxed.

Nitrous Oxide (Laughing Gas) One of the most popular of all the relaxing agents used in dentistry is nitrous oxide. Nitrous oxide was known as laughing gas in the 1800's when first used as a form of entertainment in circuses (see Chapter 1). However, in the dental office it is combined with oxygen and inhaled through a nose mask promoting a dream-like sensation, euphoria, and a feeling of well being for the anxious patient. Nitrous oxide with oxygen does not produce an unconscious state. Patients are most definitely awake but are frequently heard to say, "I know you are doing something but it really doesn't matter."

Full Mouth Surgery and Hospital Care The idea of "getting it all over with at once" may be appealing and can be accomplished in the specially equipped periodontal office or hospital operating room.

Patients are given either general anesthesia or a milder sedation, which promotes a sense of detachment and calm during the procedure. The surgical techniques themselves are the same, regardless of whether performed in segments or at one time. The full mouth procedure however may last two to four hours and would involve a more uncomfortable and slightly longer recovery period than expected of the patient having segmental surgery.

Surgery for Deep or Difficult-to-Clean Pockets

Patients with deep, difficult-to-clean pockets and/or continuing signs of inflammation (Fig. 9-1) are unable to effectively fight the accumulation of plaque and more likely to experience progression of their disease. The benefits of periodontal surgery in these cases include improved ability to perform effective plaque control, halting the continual deepening of pockets, rebuilding lost support and prevention of tooth loss.

Generally, only part of your mouth will be treated at a single sitting. If one quadrant (one quarter of the mouth) or one half of the mouth is treated, the patient can still eat comfortably and perform regular plaque control on the untreated side.

After arrival at the periodontist's office, the patient is encouraged to become as comfortable as possible in the dental chair. You can loosen your collar or belt, perhaps even remove your shoes. In addition to any relaxation options you may have chosen, a local anesthetic will be given. No pain will be felt.

The periodontist is assisted by a nurse or dental assistant who is not only trained to help technically during the procedure, but also is particularly concerned about the patient's comfort.

One or a combination of several corrective procedures will be chosen to treat the deep pockets.

Gingivectomy – Gingivoplasty

Gingivectomy is the removal of gingival or gum tissue, just as appendectomy is removal of the appendix. At one time, it was the most widely used type of periodontal surgery. This procedure reduces the depth of periodontal pockets and at the same time exposes the calculus or tartar for more effective removal. The gingivectomy may be the preferred procedure in cases of swollen gums. Gingivectomy is usually performed when there is no bone loss, and is therefore not

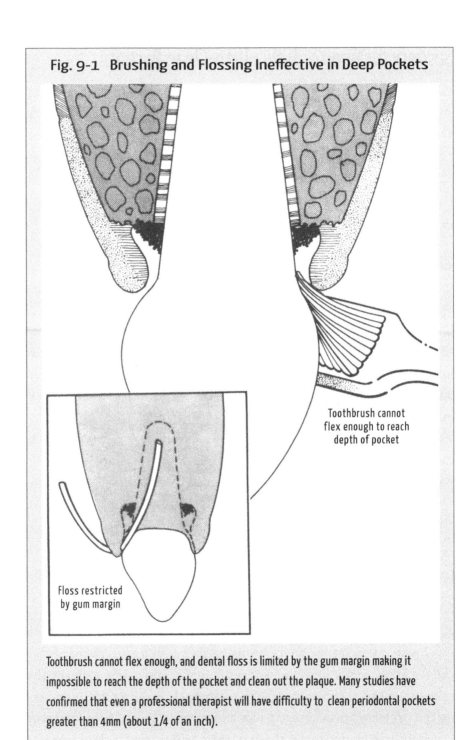

Fig. 9-1 Brushing and Flossing Ineffective in Deep Pockets

Toothbrush cannot flex enough to reach depth of pocket

Floss restricted by gum margin

Toothbrush cannot flex enough, and dental floss is limited by the gum margin making it impossible to reach the depth of the pocket and clean out the plaque. Many studies have confirmed that even a professional therapist will have difficulty to clean periodontal pockets greater than 4mm (about 1/4 of an inch).

generally employed in advanced cases. In the past, over-utilization of the gingivectomy removed much of the protective gum (gingiva) tissue. Gingivoplasty refers to the reshaping or sculpturing of the gum tissues. These minor adjustments will improve esthetics and/or enhance the ability to perform effective plaque control.

Flap Procedures

Most advanced cases of gum disease will predictably benefit from a flap procedure. As the name implies, a delicate incision separating the periodontal pockets and gum tissue from the tooth creates a flap of gum tissue. The flap may include both an inner flap consisting of the gum tissue on the tongue side of the tooth and an outer flap developed from the gum on the cheek side of the tooth. What makes this procedure special? Unlike gingivectomy where gum tissue is removed, this procedure preserves the gum tissue, which is returned to its place at the end of the surgery. Little or no gum tissue is lost.

The main advantage however, of this sophisticated flap approach is that it provides access to the underlying diseased structures. Once the incision has been made, several delicate steps will follow. The flaps are gently separated from the teeth and bone so that the meticulous step of the procedure can be accomplished: the removal of all the diseased tissue, calculus, and other pocket remnants located in the small convoluted defects within the bone.

Following thorough removal of all diseased tissue, the root surfaces are scaled and smoothed. The surgery may be completed at this point or continued with treatment of the underlying bone.

Treating Tooth Supporting Bone

Periodontitis results in formation of defects between the bone and the roots of the teeth, which become a focal area for reinfection. In many cases, treatment of the underlying bone (technically termed osseous surgery), which supports the teeth, is considered an essential part of managing advanced periodontal disease. With the flap raised and undesirable tissues removed, the bone surrounding the defects is directly visible and treatable.

Bone Reshaping This procedure reduces thick margins, which project from the bone around the teeth, and improves the positioning of the replaced flaps. Small amounts of bone around the defects and adjacent teeth may also be removed to enhance the healing and assist in reducing pockets.

Root Removal Molars, which have two or three roots, sometimes suffer bone loss between the roots known as furcation involvement (Fig. 6-4). When there is no alternative, removal of the root with the most bone loss may be elected to allow the healthier remaining part of the tooth to survive. A root canal, which involves removing the tooth's nerve and other components of the dental pulp (Fig. 2- 2) is performed either prior to or directly after this procedure. Afterwards, a crown is often recommended.

Regeneration: For New Tooth-Supporting Tissues

One of the more advanced methods for treating bone defects is known as regeneration; the growth of cells to form new tissues which replace missing or damaged ones. This process goes on naturally throughout our bodies providing replacement tissues for those that become old and die. As we age, this process becomes slower and less efficient. But usually it is still working well enough throughout our lifetime to repair our cuts and bruises.

In the past, predictable regeneration of tooth-supporting tissues (bone, root cementum, and attaching fibers) was only a dream. The periodontal defect being under constant attack by bacterial plaque, food debris and retained calculus was a difficult area to expect good results. Today, however, use of the advanced procedures discussed in this next section have turned regeneration into a reality.

Various materials can be placed into the bone defect in a fashion similar to puttying up a hole in your wall. The bone replacement graft becomes incorporated into the defect and/or replaced by the patient's own bone during healing. Bone grafting material can be acquired from a number of different sources.

Patient's Bone   The patient's own bone is an excellent and convenient grafting material. Bits of bone shavings collected during periodontal surgery can be placed directly into the bone defects. A recent extraction space or other areas of the mouth can also be excellent sources of graft material.

Human or Animal Origin   Bone can be procured from companies specializing in supplying these materials and can ensure that the source bone undergoes vigorous screening, testing and special techniques to eradicate the possibility of disease or infection transmission. This bone is used alone or mixed with the patient's own bone, as a combined grafting material.

Bone Substitutes and Tissue Stimulating Proteins   Synthetic materials may also be placed into the bone defect. These substances can act (in a manner similar to human or animal bone grafts) as a filler to maintain space for regeneration, or serve principally to stimulate the growth of new bone and attachment.

Tissue stimulating proteins (usually in gel-like form) are substances that can be placed in the bone defect and along the root surfaces to encourage the growth of new bone and biological attachment to the root.

Membranes

Regeneration techniques often incorporate a membrane either alone or in combination with bone grafting, in a process called guided tissue regeneration, in order to separate the tissues we want to grow (in this case, bone and fiber attachments) from the gum and other soft tissues.

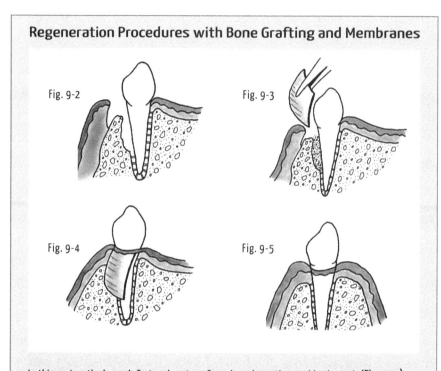

Regeneration Procedures with Bone Grafting and Membranes

Fig. 9-2

Fig. 9-3

Fig. 9-4

Fig. 9-5

In this series, the bone defect and root surfaces have been thoroughly cleaned. (Fig. 9-2) A bone substitute or graft material is placed, while a self-dissolving membrane is prepared (Fig. 9-3) and then draped over the area (Fig. 9-4) Within three months, new bone and possible attachments seen in (Fig. 9-5) can be expected to replace a substantial part of the previous defect.

By covering the defect, the membrane can promote regeneration by acting as a filter, which contains the graft within the defect (Fig. 9-2 - 9-5). Membranes are made of various materials. Some are self-dissolving, while others require a second surgical procedure to be removed.

Influencing Successful Regeneration

The overall success of regeneration techniques has been very promising. The factors which influence the success of these procedures include the materials used, the type of defects treated, the control of risk factors, such as smoking, and the surgeon's ability and experience.

Cosmetic Periodontal Surgery

The mouth is the most expressive part of you face. Sadness, fear, exultation and allure are all remarkably communicated to someone via the mouth.

Few things are more pleasing to the eye than a beautiful smile. A beautiful smile radiates health, vitality, warmth and yes, sex appeal. Cosmetic periodontal surgery procedures correct problems in the relationship between the teeth, gum and surrounding tissues that often are the cause of an unattractive smile.

Smile Consultation It may be surprising to discover just how many esthetics problems in the mouth can be resolved after consulting with a periodontist. Looking at your smile together, you and the periodontist can review the specific procedures that will enable you to achieve the smile you always wanted.

Crown Lengthening: Correcting "Short" Teeth

An individual may appear to have short teeth only to discover that the teeth are of normal length, but burdened with an abundance of gum tissue, sometimes referred to as a "gummy smile." These patients have suffered for years, hiding their teeth due to embarrassment, either because they thought their teeth were too small or showed too much gum while smiling. The benefits of cosmetic surgery (gingivectomy or a flap procedure) are immediate and dramatic as the full natural, attractive smile is revealed. See the opposite page story on "Short Teeth Shirley".

Crown lengthening increases tooth length. The word "crown" refers to that part of the tooth normally present above the gum line. Although crown lengthening is often required to increase the length of the tooth for esthetics, your dentist may also prescribe this treatment when the available tooth structure is too short or there is not enough tooth structure required for your dentist to prepare for caps or crowns.

Gum Replacement Grafts

For Weak Gums and Exposed Roots Gum recession and its associated root exposure can be very unpleasant especially when it appears in the front of the mouth. Exposed roots can also make an individual look older than one's real age, as well as lead to sensitivity and cavities. In addition, when the quality of the gum is poor, these fragile tissues can become easily inflamed or damaged from injury leading to root exposure.

Techniques for grafting gum or compatible soft tissues within the mouth have made it possible to reinforce areas of weak gum tissues and frequently cover exposed roots. Gum grafts may also be indicated to strengthen gum tissues associated with planed crowns, bridges and orthodontic treatment.

Pedicle Grafts remain partially attached to the patient's own gum tissue and are therefore limited to close proximity defects.

Free Grafts are completely detached from their source and can be utilized anywhere in the mouth. Free grafts are usually procured from the palate. Gum grafts are also available from companies that specialize in animal or human grafts (same as with the bone) and fall under the "free" category as they were not attached to the patients' oral tissues.

Short Teeth Shirley

Shirley, though an attractive 25-year-old woman, was extremely self-conscious about her "short" teeth. In fact, she was so disturbed by them that Shirley would automatically cover her mouth with her hands whenever she smiled. Why? Because she was embarrassed when people would always say, "your teeth are so small", "you have such a gummy smile". After examining her mouth and a new set of x-rays, I was able to advise Shirley that in fact her teeth weren't small, just covered by excess gum tissue. This condition where gum tissues cover parts of the tooth often occurs when, during the natural eruption of the teeth, the gum line fails to retract to its normal position.

Immediately after performing the crown-lengthening procedure, nearly 30% of her teeth that had been previously submerged under her gums became visible. Her teeth were now much more natural (both in shape and size) contributing to a proud, gorgeous new smile.

And now when she proudly shows off those pearly whites, it's with no hands!!

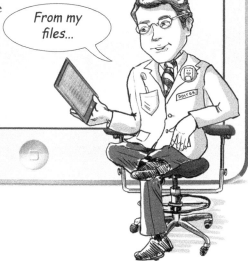

From my files...

Repairing Gum Indentations

Unsightly indentations in the gums may occur after tooth removal or as a result of accident or diseases. These defects themselves are not only disfiguring but cause the replacement tooth to be out of proportion and unattractive in comparison with the remaining teeth. Special techniques are utilized to repair and fill in these types of esthetic defects by combining gum and bone grafting procedures.

Frenectomy

The frenum is composed of fibers extending from the lip and cheek to the gums. Frenum can contribute to recession of the gum margin, root exposure and pain during normal brushing. A frenum attached too closely to the gum margin can open the walls of an existing periodontal pocket during talking and eating, and retard good healing following surgery. In these situations, removal of the frenum or frenectomy is recommended. There is no harm in being without a frenum. A frenectomy is often incorporated with other surgical techniques or during orthodontic treatment to aid in the movement of teeth and enhance their stability.

Concluding Procedures and Follow Up Care

The following procedures are generally performed at the conclusion of surgery.

Replacement of Flaps and Suturing   The replaced flaps or grafted tissues are sutured (sewed) to maintain the flaps in position. Some sutures are removed during a post-operative visit while others, made of biodegradable material, are self-dissolving.

Periodontal Dressing   A periodontal dressing may be used. This surgical dressing is a mixture of materials that have the initial consistency of putty. It is easily shaped around the surgery area and between the teeth. The dressing can help protect the surgical site from inadvertent trauma during eating or tooth brushing. Within a few minutes, the dressing becomes firm and will be removed at a later visit.

Post-Operative Instructions   Post-operative instructions contain important information about how to care for your mouth after surgery, such as where and how to brush, recommended foods to eat and the telephone number to call with any questions. You will receive a prescription for the relief of any discomfort, as well as antibiotics and a medicated mouth rinse if appropriate for the procedure.

Patients usually return in a week to ten days for their first post operative visit, which includes examination, removal of any periodontal dressing and sutures (if they are not self-dissolving), special oral hygiene instructions and other procedures that may assist the healing process.

Discomfort   For the record, let us face the question of discomfort head on. Yes, the surgical procedure may be unpleasant, but it is not painful. Today, besides the possible annoyance of the anesthetic needle, the only real discomfort is having to hold your mouth open long enough and wide enough to complete the treatment.

After the anesthetic wears off, you may experience somewhat of a sore mouth and possibly minor swelling. However, with medication, the discomfort is considerably minimized. Many patients are back to normal activities the following day. Soreness can occasionally last a bit longer for some, depending on the exact nature and extent of the surgery.

Changes in the Mouth after Periodontal Surgery

With successful periodontal surgery, many welcome changes occur in the gum tissues, including reduced pockets and elimination of active inflammation, as well as a clean, fresh feeling in the mouth. Other changes, generally as a result of flap or gingivectomy surgery, may be of concern to the patient at first and are described in the following segment.

■ Movement of Gum Line

Sometimes the gum line heals farther away from its position prior to surgery. This is the result of eliminating diseased materials that created an infected layer between the gum and the bone. After surgery, the healthy gum lays above the bone without any interposed infected tissue. In the front of the mouth, surgical procedures can be modified to avoid or reduce the shift of the gum line.

■ Food Catches

As a result of the change in the gum line, food previously collected within the gum pockets will now be found between the top of the gum and the tooth itself. Patients often refer to this area as "spaces between the teeth." The food is now exposed and easily accessible for cleaning... a far better situation than existed previously when trapped food particles quietly contributed to gum disease.

■ Tooth Sensitivity

During the first weeks after periodontal surgery, patients may notice sensitivity to certain foods and temperature extremes along the teeth. Generally this sensitivity will diminish over time. If sensitivity continues, it can usually be remedied by application of various medications and desensitizing toothpastes.

■ Loose Teeth

Immediately following surgery, the teeth may seem looser than previously. This is normal. The teeth will tighten to at least the same degree of firmness as before surgery, and often firmer. If teeth are still loose after treatment because of extensive bone loss or trauma, splinting techniques are used to join weak teeth to adjacent firmer teeth making one strong combined unit. Splinting methods vary from the use of reinforced glue or bonding, to crowning and joining together the teeth to be splinted.

All Things Considered The majority of patients see these inconveniences as minor annoyances along the road to saving their teeth. Especially when one considers that a patient who refuses surgery may experience recurrent abscesses, sore gums, loose teeth, expensive dental treatment to support failing teeth, and ultimately the loss of their teeth.

Success of Periodontal Surgery

The long-term success rate in periodontal surgery is excellent, with studies over many years showing that patients who completed this treatment have kept most, if not all of their teeth. The earlier in the stage of periodontal disease that treatment is started, the less surgery is required.

It is definitely to the patient's advantage to seek a consulation, as early as possible, with a dental professional. Indeed, even when periodontitis is advanced, surgery offers a very real hope for the continued longevity and enjoyment of your natural teeth.

Who Should Not Have Periodontal Surgery?

Occasionally, patients with significant periodontal disease may not be good surgery candidates for the following reasons:

Unwilling to Fully Commit to Oral Hygiene Patients who are not motivated to develop a basic regimen of preventive oral hygiene are not candidates for surgery. Even after successful treatment, there is no immunity from gum disease. It can return without good plaque control and regular visits to the periodontist.

Medical Complications Medical problems such as unstable diabetes, compromised immunity, or bleeding disorders may contraindicate surgery. Patients, who are pregnant, undergoing extreme stress, are severely debilitated, psychologically impaired or who have had a recent heart attack, require special consideration prior to surgery. Surgery is not performed on patients who are uncontrolled alcoholics or drug abusers.

Patient Medications Certain medications can cause an altered reaction to surgery and may need to be adjusted with the physician's cooperation in order to proceed with surgery. These medications include blood thinners, antidepressants, thyroid replacements, steroids and various cancer drugs.

Teeth with Hopeless Prognosis If supporting bone deterioration has progressed so far that even the most advanced procedures cannot repair the devastating results of periodontal disease, a hopeless situation exists. The tooth or teeth should be removed.

Alternatives to Surgery in Advanced Disease

In advanced periodontal disease, modern surgery is an efficient and predictable means of reducing pocket depths, eliminating periodontal disease and ultimately keeping your natural teeth.

The following alternatives however, may be presented to you for consideration.

Scaling, Root Planing and Oral Hygiene Only

These initial therapy procedures may be suggested as an alternative to periodontal surgery, and are sometimes referred to as soft tissue management. The support for this approach is based on the theory that with meticulous plaque control, a stable periodontal condition can be established and further loss of support for the tooth avoided. In order to maximize the effects of this approach, frequent professional office visits may be required, depending on the patient's ability to control plaque accumulation. These treatments may need to be scheduled every few weeks to a few months, depending on the patient's level of plaque control. While the scientific basis for this approach is sound, the practicality is another matter. If patients present for their appointments as often as required and plaque control is maintained, this approach can be beneficial. However, having patients come in very frequently is not as easy as it may seem. Experience shows that even with the best intentions of the patient (and the dentist) this alternative to surgery more often than not falls short of reaching its goal.

Medications

Various medications and solutions have been recommended to resolve gum problems including antibiotics, anti-inflammatory agents, antiseptics, mixtures of baking soda, salt and peroxide, mouthwashes and saltwater rinses. Some medications are taken systemically (such as antibiotics) while others are placed directly into the pockets incorporating special time-releasing substances. Some toothpastes contain ingredients that can reduce gingivitis. While certain solutions or drugs, especially antibiotics, are recommended to supplement the treatment of gum disease, to date there is limited evidence for the efficacy of any of these materials as a predictable stand-alone replacement therapy in advanced disease.

A Combination Approach: The Best Alternative

When the surgery option has been contraindicated, needs to be postponed or is declined by the patient, a combination of scaling and root planing along with medications is likely to be the most effective alternative measure prescribed by the periodontist for deep, difficult-to-clean periodontal pockets and unresolved signs of inflammation. The primary goal will be to slow the disease from advancing. The major limitation to the success of all the described alternatives to surgery is that reaching and thoroughly cleaning the pockets with scaling, root planing and/or medications is extremely difficult, even in the hands of the most skillful professionals. There is simply a problem with physical access to the plaque-affected areas (Fig. 9-1).

Most studies have shown that deeper pockets are more likely to progress and infect deeper structures supporting the teeth. In addition, while there may be an initial improvement with these methods, maintaining the results over a long-term have proven to be an additional challenge.

Some Have Beaten the Odds And yet, given all these limitations, there are patients in nearly every periodontal practice who, did not have surgical therapy for their deep pockets, have beaten the odds and were successful in keeping their teeth by participating in an alternative combination approach utilizing medications, scaling and root planing.

The majority of these patients have shown a strong commitment to performing excellent oral hygiene at home and consistently presenting for the prescribed periodontal maintenance visits. In addition, these dedicated patients understand that their periodontal pockets may never be completely reduced. Therefore, during the course of their treatment, when areas of the mouth become sensitive or demonstrate acute infections, modifications of the treatment protocol, including changes in the medication regimen or localized surgery may be required.

While achieving success for teeth's deep pockets with alternative therapy is a challenge, the dental literature has demonstrated reduction in pocket depths and gum inflammation in a number of clinical studies. This is especially noteworthy when the disease is localized in the mouth or associated with teeth toward the front of the mouth that have only one root.

Too Many Options?

Sometimes the many treatment options can be confusing. You should speak candidly with an experienced dentist or periodontist to discuss the advantages and disadvantages of each of the various therapies.

10

Dental Implants

Modern Solutions
for Missing Teeth

Replacing Missing Teeth

Generally, missing teeth (other than wisdom teeth) should be replaced in order to balance the biting pressures, retain chewing efficiency and maintain the position of the remaining teeth in your mouth. The replacements will stabilize the mouth by keeping contact between teeth and reducing the possibility of shifting and rotation. At one time, replacements necessitated damage to healthy remaining teeth for support. If the patient was totally toothless, he or she would suffer the potential embarrassment of ill-fitting dentures.

Now, there is an alternative to the age-old solutions of toothless spaces: predictable dental implants. Just as with other body parts, teeth can be replaced with implant-supported prostheses (substitute artificial teeth). The result is a natural-looking improvement in your ability to talk, eat and smile with confidence.

Types of Dental Implants Dental implants are usually made of the same biocompatible, titanium metal used in many other types of implants throughout the body. The dental implant replaces the tooth root, and is connected to different prostheses that serve as substitutes for missing teeth. The two major categories of implants are endosseous that are placed within the jawbone and subperiosteal that is placed on the bone just below the gum.

Implants are Like Teeth

Most implants in use today are endosseous or placed in the bone (about 1/2 to 3/4 inch). Because they are similar in appearance and size to the tooth root being replaced, this type of implant is also referred to as a root form implant. The implants usually have a threaded surface like a screw (Fig. 10-1) and may contain small vents or holes. The texture of the dental implant's outer surface can be smooth, machine roughened, coated or any combination thereof.

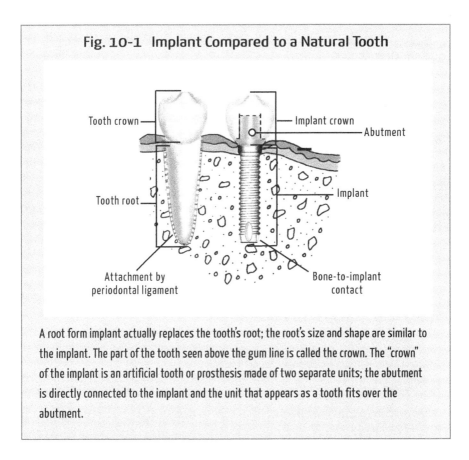

Fig. 10-1 Implant Compared to a Natural Tooth

Tooth crown

Implant crown

Abutment

Tooth root

Implant

Attachment by periodontal ligament

Bone-to-implant contact

A root form implant actually replaces the tooth's root; the root's size and shape are similar to the implant. The part of the tooth seen above the gum line is called the crown. The "crown" of the implant is an artificial tooth or prosthesis made of two separate units; the abutment is directly connected to the implant and the unit that appears as a tooth fits over the abutment.

Once the implant becomes firmly attached to the surrounding bone, an extension-base is added to the implant (abutment) on which the artificial tooth or prosthesis is placed.

Advantages Over Traditional Tooth Replacements

Instead of Altering Healthy Teeth to Make a Fixed Bridge

A fixed bridge is a traditional method for replacing missing teeth especially in small spaces where natural teeth are present on either side. The bridge is formed by connecting crowns (caps), that slip over altered teeth on either side of the toothless space, to a middle false tooth or teeth. The main disadvantage of the traditional bridge is that healthy natural teeth have to be shaved down to fit the connecting crowns.

Instead of shaving down healthy teeth to accommodate a bridge, a single dental implant is placed in the toothless space. Not only does it save the tooth on either side from being ground down to a very small stump, but it also eliminates the need for having to do root canal treatment, which is often required on teeth being prepared to receive a crown.

If more than one tooth is missing, several implants can be placed. The artificial teeth are then securely fitted to the implants with either tiny screws or cement; they cannot be removed by the patient. The implant alternative has many advantages including the look and feel of natural teeth, preserving the health of the remaining teeth and more efficient plaque control.

In Place of Removable Partial Dentures

Removable partial dentures are constructed on a metal frame, covered by a gum-simulating plastic, which holds the artificial teeth. This type of prosthesis is supported by a combination of the toothless

Guess Whose Coming to Dinner: Grandma Sarah

Grandma Sarah is a vibrant 88-year old lady determined to enjoy life to the maximum and not accustomed to complaining. But during dinner, Grandma would spend a lot of time cutting up her food. And to make things worse, her dentures always seemed to be moving around in her mouth. The constant clicking sound of the unstable dentures was embarrassing to her and uncomfortable for the rest the family. During our visit, Sarah confided that she was humiliated about the instability of her false teeth, but unable to talk about it with the family.

I demonstrated that based on her x-rays, six implants in her lower jaw would easily hold the denture in her mouth, secure and stable throughout chewing, eating and talking. I explained that I would be using a technique that allows the placement of implants to be followed by the immediate insertion of a new denture. Three weeks later, Sarah left my office to meet the family for dinner at a local restaurant, literally within hours of having completed the treatment. The celebratory meal with her family was the most enjoyable in a long time (and quieter).

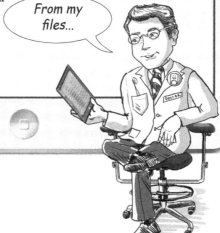

From my files...

ridge and the remaining teeth via metal clasps or other attachments. Patients may report that partial dentures are like having a "mouthful of hardware," are difficult to wear and feel unnatural. Sometimes, pressure from the partial denture attachments can weaken the natural teeth.

As an alternative, a fixed or permanent-type prosthesis can be made with implants placed in the position of the missing teeth. In effect, this solution is an expanded version of the individual implant technique described previously. When more than one tooth is missing, implants can be utilized to anchor an implant-supported bridge.

To Add Support and Stability to Removable Full Dentures

A removable full denture replaces all the natural teeth and therefore is completely dependent on the toothless jaw for support and stability. While some patients have successfully worn removable full dentures, many complain about feeling self-conscious due to dentures wobbling, clicking and pain, as well as loss of taste and poor eating ability. An implant-denture can help in one of two ways:

Fixed Implant Denture   With an adequate number of implants, a fixed-implant denture, secured by screws or cement to the implants, will restore the feeling and function similar to the natural set of teeth. This prosthesis can not be removed by the patient. A dental professional however, may periodically remove the prosthesis for examination (see story about Grandma Sarah on previous page).

Removable Implant Denture   If a fixed solution is not possible, an implant-retained denture will dramatically increase the stability and confidence in wearing a traditional full denture. The implants, acting as anchors, are connected to the denture by hidden attachments. This type of prosthesis is removed by the patient for inspection and cleaning at home.

The Dental Implant Procedure

The Implant Team An excellent approach to coordinating the placement of dental implants and the final prosthesis (artificial teeth) is the implant team that allows patients to benefit from the special expertise of each team member. The implant team works closely to coordinate the various aspects of the implant therapy.

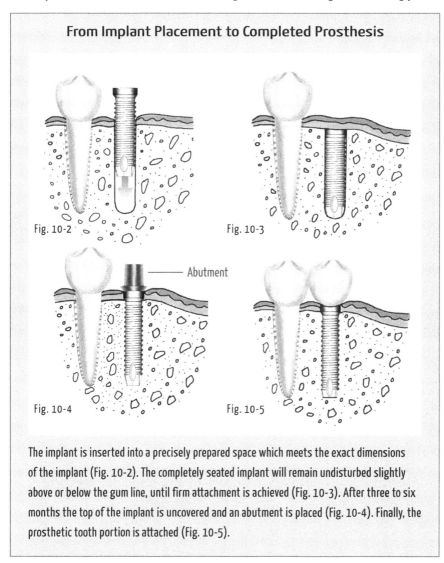

From Implant Placement to Completed Prosthesis

Fig. 10-2

Fig. 10-3

— Abutment

Fig. 10-4

Fig. 10-5

The implant is inserted into a precisely prepared space which meets the exact dimensions of the implant (Fig. 10-2). The completely seated implant will remain undisturbed slightly above or below the gum line, until firm attachment is achieved (Fig. 10-3). After three to six months the top of the implant is uncovered and an abutment is placed (Fig. 10-4). Finally, the prosthetic tooth portion is attached (Fig. 10-5).

The patient is usually unaware of the extensive consultations that often transpire between team members prior to and after the actual implant procedure. The results however, of this professional cooperation, will help to ensure the correct treatment plan for each individual and contribute to the overall success of the implant.

A periodontist, the recognized expert in the gum and bone tissues that surround and support the implant, routinely performs a wide variety of sophisticated surgical procedures. This combination of knowledge and skill makes the periodontal specialist an excellent choice to be the surgical member of the team to place your implants.

Of course, there are dentists who are not specialists in periodontics, but are qualified to place implants based on their experience and advanced studies. Choosing the right surgeon to place your implants is an important decision and should not be taken lightly.

The prosthetic aspect (placing the crowns) is completed by a dentist experienced in implant prostheses. This will likely be your general dentist. If he or she does not perform implant prostheses or if your mouth is particularly complicated, you will be referred to someone with the necessary skill and understanding.

Getting Started The preparatory steps prior to implant placement are similar to periodontal surgery including a thorough medical and dental history, oral exam, x-rays and possibly plaster molds of your teeth. The molds may be used by your dentist to create a surgical template which guides the periodontist when placing the implants. The use of more detailed radiographs such as CT x-ray may be recommended to enhance the evaluation of the surgical site with 3-d imagery.

A consultation with all members of the implant team will take place to coordinate each stage of the treatment.

Implants: Step by Step

First Stage: Implant Placement

The anesthesia and relaxation techniques are similar to periodontal surgery. In this case, a flap is made and the implant receptor site fashioned in the bone to precisely accommodate the implant's dimensions. The implant is then either gently pushed or rotated into the prepared site (Fig. 10-1).

The surgery will be completed with suturing and a review of post-operative instructions, not unlike periodontal surgery. After the implant surgery however, patients with removable dentures may have to leave them out of their mouths for a short period. Additional dietary limitations may be prescribed. Return visits will be scheduled for check-ups and, if required, suture removal. The implants remain undisturbed either below or just above the gum tissues to promote the firm attachment needed between implant and bone (Fig. 10-3). A temporary bridge or denture may be worn during this period in place of the missing teeth.

Second Stage: Preparation for Prosthesis

After approximately three to six months, if the top of the implant is not protruding through the gum, a small opening is made by the periodontist to reveal the top of the implant. This is a relatively short procedure performed with local anesthesia. A protective cover or an immediate abutment is then placed on the implant.

Third Stage: Placement of the Prosthesis

The dentist will remove the protective cover to access the inner implant area and permit attachment of those parts that will form the prosthesis or artificial tooth. These parts include the abutment that attaches directly to the implant and the prosthetic crown (artificial tooth) or denture. All implant parts are made to fit the exact size and shape of the implant your periodontist placed during the first stage. The final texture, size, color and shape of the replacement prosthesis will be designed to blend with any remaining natural teeth and your general facial features.

One Stage Option: Immediate Implant and Crown

"Teeth in an Hour" and "One Day Implants and Crowns" are expressions frequently used in advertisements to describe the situation where the implant is placed, and immediately a crown is inserted, so the patient walks out of the office with a completed restoration in one sitting. While this technique is very appealing, it is not always possible to perform. Many limitations including presence of infections, lack of adequate bone, consideration of the patient's bite, the condition of the remaining teeth, as well as the position in the mouth of the intended implant, will all have a significant influence on the recommendation of the surgeon to perform this technique.

Augmentation – For Improved Implant Success

Previously, a lack of adequate quality or quantity of bone meant a patient could not have implants placed or were forced to be placed in less than ideal positioning. Today however, augmentation procedures can enhance areas of deficient bone and improve positioning of the implant. These procedures usually require bone grafting and membrane placement. The rate of success is good. However, the waiting period before the prosthesis can be attached may be extended from six to twelve months.

Situations that may benefit from the use of these special procedures include the following:

Thin or Defective Jaw Bones Jaws that are too thin, deformed or have been damaged as a result of an accident or disease, can be repaired and enlarged.

During Tooth Removal Hopeless teeth may be removed and an implant placed immediately. Sometimes, only augmentation is possible at the time of tooth removal to prepare the area for a future implant.

Sinus Proximity The sinus is an air passage that rests within the bone area at about the level of your cheek just below the eye socket. A common limitation to implant therapy in the back of the upper jaw is a low sinus, i.e. the sinus is too close to the implant area. To solve this problem, the lower part of the sinus is raised and replaced with grafted material (sinus lift) allowing implants to be placed.

When Dental Implants May Not Be Advisable

Other than not having the adequate quality and quantity of bone, there are additional considerations that could limit or contraindicate recommending dental implants.

Medical Condition Any medical condition or medications that might influence the patient's ability to have periodontal surgery will be of equal concern to the implant patient and the periodontist.

Smoking Smoking can jeopardize the success of implants. The patient's willingness to stop or reduce smoking should be addressed prior to the decision to have implants.

Gum Disease Implants are not placed in a mouth with untreated, active gum disease. The gum infection can contribute to the failure of the most skillfully placed implants. With certain exceptions, such as in conjunction with tooth removal, periodontal disease must be under control prior to implant therapy.

Poor Oral Hygiene Oral hygiene must be adequate to assure that the gums around the implants stay healthy. The remaining natural teeth must also be kept as free as possible from plaque build-up and food debris.

Peri-Implant Diseases

Peri-implant diseases are inflammatory conditions affecting the soft and hard oral tissues around dental implants. Similar to a natural tooth, bacteria can build up on the implant, above and below the gum line. Over time, the bacteria irritate the gum tissue, causing it to become inflamed, damaging the tissue and if not caught early, causing the bone structure supporting the implant to deteriorate. Peri-implant infections may be successfully treated and are reversible if caught early. However, if the deterioration reaches the bone supporting the dental implant, surgical intervention may be required.

Risks

The possibility that an implant will not "take" is small, but nevertheless exists. If an implant should not be successful, a replacement implant can often be inserted. Rare problems, such as temporary or extended loss of sensation or infection can occur when usually distant nerves or other anatomical areas are involved. In the event that your periodontist anticipates an area of special concern, a full explanation of these matters will be added to the thorough discussion of the risks and benefits that precedes the placement of any dental implant.

Dental Implant Success

Fortunately, studies around the world confirm that tested and approved implant systems used by well-trained therapists yield high rates of success. No longer must patients suffer the discomfort and humiliation of unstable and awkward traditional tooth replacements. Instead, they can start enjoying the many benefits of modern dental implants including a natural, secure smile with confident, comfortable eating and speech.

11

Periodontal Maintenance

Keeping Your Healthy Smile

Ensuring Results of Treatment

The potential for infection and pocket formation in the treated patient is as great as before the patient had periodontal disease. There is one important difference: the periodontal patient has already demonstrated a susceptibility to gum disease and therefore may have a recurrent problem. A vigorous monitored program to ensure a clean mouth with minimal plaque is essential to ensure the results of your treatment and to quickly identify any changes or reinfection that could preceed a return to gum disease. For patients who have had implants, the concern is the same, as bacteria and conditions that cause gum disease could mean serious problems for the implants as well.

Determining the Maintenance Schedule

Periodontists provide a program of reevaluation and treatment visits, termed supportive periodontal therapy, periodontal maintenance or just maintenance. Maintenance treatments begin soon after completion of active therapy and are carefully planned to accommodate the unique needs of each patient.

Studies have demonstrated that a minimum of two to three months between maintenance visits will generally significantly reduce the chances of the return of gum disease. During the first year, however following active treatment, the patient's plaque control ability will often fluctuate while establishing acceptable intervals between maintenance visits. This is because patients require time to establish a safe period during which plaque can be adequately controlled. During this period, a patient's visits may be as frequent as bi-weekly or monthly. The frequency will be influenced by:

- Severity of the periodontal disease
- Type of treatment that was rendered
- Number of implants placed and type of prosthesis
- Results of treatment
- Effectiveness of the patient's personal plaque control
- Type of restorative treatments (bridges, crowns etc.)

Sometimes, when the gum disease is mild, the periodontist and general dentist alternate maintenance visits.

Most specialists and general dentists employ certified dental hygienists who play a major role in providing maintenance care,

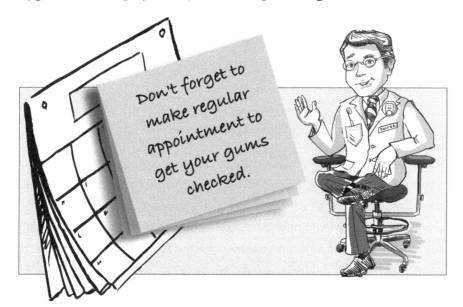

under the doctors' supervision and guidance. Dental hygienists have enhanced experience and knowledge in the special requirements of periodontal patients.

Periodontal Maintenance Treatments

Periodontal maintenance treatments will include many of the following services during each visit:

- Review all aspects of the completed treatment
- Monitor areas with special problems
- Update medical status and medication regimen
- Check for bleeding and mobility
- Probe periodontal pockets
- Test to identify areas of suspected bacterial involvement
- Review oral hygiene techniques and plaque control aids
- Remove plaque and tartar – scaling
- Smooth root surfaces – root planing
- Polish and whiten the teeth
- Evaluate the bite to ensure balance and comfort
- Assess the effectiveness of the bite guard
- Reduce sensitivity, if noted
- Evaluate health of dental implants
- Prescribe medications as needed

General Dentist's Role During Maintenance

Even though your general dentist will likely be kept up-to-date with your progress during maintenance, and advised of any problems that need attention, he or she is still responsible for your overall dental health. At least annual examinations are required to evaluate for new or recurrent decay, replace missing fillings and worn crowns, as well as an overall check-up of your mouth.

Periodic X-Rays

During the course of long-term maintenance therapy, you can expect to have x-rays taken periodically to assess the bone stability around the teeth, development of dental decay and other abnormalities. Implants are usually x-rayed during the first year, and depending on the situation, every one or two years thereafter.

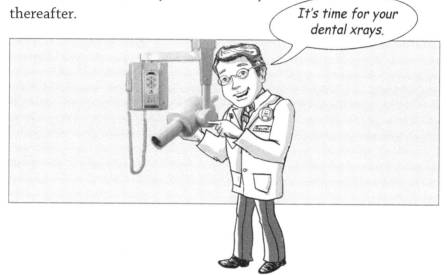

It's time for your dental xrays.

Smoking Cessation Programs

Due to the universal acceptance of smoking's influence on poor oral health, you can be certain that when you are ready to stop smoking, your periodontist will be ready to help. This may be via a referral to a smoking-cessation program in your area, or the periodontal office may have its own stop-smoking program.

Maintenance...an Excellent Investment

Susceptible periodontal patients, who are committed to a regular maintenance program, will significantly reduce their chances of further gum disease. But even if there should be adverse changes in the health of their gums, the problems can be caught at an early stage when intervention is usually simple and predictable. And don't forget, early detection almost always means saving money.

A maintenance program, under the careful supervision of a periodontist, is probably as close as a patient can get to an insurance policy against advancing and recurrent periodontal disease. Once you start, stick to it. You will be glad you did!

12

I'm Glad You Asked

Answers to patients'
most common questions
about Gum Disease
and Dental Implants

How Much Will My Treatments Cost?

It's not facetious to say that the cost of periodontal therapy can range from a few dollars to more than ten thousand dollars for all four quadrants of the mouth with comprehensive care, including bone grafting and other advanced treatments. By investing in a good toothbrush and dental floss, a patient can reverse and cure the early stages of gum disease. The more sophisticated techniques required to treat advanced disease demand greater skill and knowledge on the part of the specialist, and therefore a more significant investment.

Remember that the implant procedure is usually comprised of separate stages. The first and second stages, which are surgical, may incur a cost similar to a segment of periodontal surgery, plus the added expenditure for placing the implant, and any special associated procedures. The third stage, performed by your dentist, is similar to the cost of a non-implant supported prosthesis, in addition to the cost of the connections from the implant to the prosthesis.

I Have Dental Insurance, Will It Help Pay for My Treatment?

There are many different insurance plans providing a wide range of dental benefits, some of which include periodontics and dental implants. In general, a request for a "pre-determination of benefits" of the anticipated treatment is sent to the insurance company, in order to ascertain the amount of assistance you can expect to receive.

Is Periodontal (Gum) Disease Hereditary?

A predisposition or susceptibility to gum disease may be inherited. That is, if your parents or grandparents lost their teeth due to periodontal disease, sensitivity to plaque that may result in periodontal disease could be passed on to their offspring. Certain types of periodontal disease such as aggressive periodontitis (see Chapter 3) seem to be more likely inherited.

The development of genetic profiling now makes it possible to identify certain patients with increased susceptibility. However, even with a predisposition to periodontal disease, a highly motivated patient, who observes daily rigorous plaque control, can usually ward off the loss of teeth.

Let's talk...

Your therapist will want to know when you have questions. For some, the most convenient way to discuss your questions with the doctor is by phone, others prefer face-to-face during office visits, while some practices encourage patients to send in their questions by email and avoid having to wait for an appointment or a doctor call back.

Does Periodontal Treatment or Implant Placement Hurt?

The answer to this question depends on the patient's threshold of pain and the therapist's skill. Use of appropriate instruments will reduce discomfort during scaling and root planing procedures. Periodontal surgery and implant placement are performed under local anesthesia, and therefore should be painless. Afterwards, proper use of post-operative medication and adherence to the periodontist's recommendations will reduce the likelihood of post treatment problems.

In any surgical procedure, it is important that patients consult with their therapist at the first hint of any problems or concern. An early call can lead to a speedy solution and avoid unnecessary discomfort.

Is Periodontal Disease Contagious?

Research has shown that periodontal disease (specifically gingivitis and periodontitis) is caused by the inflammatory reaction to bacteria around and within the gums, so periodontal disease technically may not be contagious. However, the bacteria that lead to the formation of inflammatory-reactive substances can be transmitted via the saliva. If family members have periodontal disease, it makes sense to avoid saliva contact by not sharing eating utensils or toothbrushes. If you notice that someone has the warning signs of periodontal problem (see opening page of Chapter 3), you may want to suggest that they see the periodontist or family dentist for an exam.

If I Have Periodontal Disease, am I Likely to Develop a Lot of Decay?

The bacteria that cause periodontal diseases are generally different from those, which cause tooth decay. Therefore, it is possible for a patient to have a mouth free of decay or fillings and still have advanced periodontal disease. The opposite is also true. Patients with numerous fillings and new decay at every office visit frequently demonstrate no evidence of gum disease or bone loss.

Unfortunately, many patients tend to regard the lack of "cavities" as a general statement that their mouth is in top shape. This of course cannot be assumed; periodontal disease and dental decay are two different problems.

How Common is Gum Disease?

Actually, it is one of most common diseases known to man. Seven out of ten adults in the world will develop gum disease at some time in their lives.

Do Children Have Gum Problems?

According to recent statistics, over 40% of all children have at least the earliest form of gum disease called gingivitis. In addition, some youngsters suffer from a very destructive form of gum disease known as aggressive periodontitis. Often times this type of periodontal disease is silent and only discovered during routine dental examination of the patient's mouth or x-rays. The treatment of children's periodontal disease is essential in order to ensure that they are able to maintain a healthy mouth for a lifetime. That's why, among other reasons, it is very important for all children to see their dentist at least twice a year.

How Long Does it Take to Complete Treatment?

Generally, patients with early gingivitis will require several visits over the course of a month to return their mouth to a healthy state. If the problems are more advanced, a complete series of periodontal treatments, including surgery, could take from three to six months or longer. The severity of the periodontal disease and approach to surgery (i.e. treating smaller or larger segments at each visit) will be a major factor influencing the duration of treatment.

Most implants require a waiting period of three to six months after surgical insertion before placement of the implant-supported prosthesis (crown, bridge or denture).

What about a Second Opinion?

Patients, who, after talking with their therapist, are uncertain about a recommendation regarding treatment, should most definitely seek a second opinion. Often the second opinion is sought after patients have been told that "everything is O.K.," despite the feeling that something seems wrong with their mouth. Patients may feel uneasy about asking for a second opinion for fear that their dentist will be insulted or resentful.

There is no cause to be concerned. An ethical professional would not hesitate to cooperate with a patient who wishes to seek another opinion. All specialists are accustomed to giving second opinions. This is neither good nor bad. It's a phenomenon of life. A second opinion may give the patient another point of view or simply confirm the first recommendation, providing the extra level of confidence needed to begin therapy.

To help you get the most from a second opinion, you should receive a written report that includes the following information:

- Diagnosis
- Treatment plan
- Prognosis for the teeth
- Complications that may affect your treatment
- Expectation regarding maintenance or follow-up care
- Cost of the treatment

Why Does Floss Get Caught Between my Teeth?

Many patients complain that their floss doesn't pass easily between teeth, especially back ones. Usually the cause is fillings with uneven edges known as overhangs (Fig. 6-2). This can occur when fillings have cracked or frayed leaving irregular surfaces. Catches can also occur around crowns (caps) whose margins do not precisely fit the tooth. All areas where dental floss does not pass smoothly along the teeth are niches for bacterial plaque to colonize. The defective fillings or crowns should be repaired or replaced.

Can Antibiotics Be Used Instead of other Treatment?

Antibiotics, both systemic and locally applied, may be utilized as adjunctive therapy in certain forms of periodontal disease. Antibiotics may also be prescribed after surgery or to treat acute infections for a short period. However, routine use of long term (potentially life saving) antibiotics as a stand-alone treatment has only limited applications in treating periodontal disease.

Who Should Perform Periodontal and Implant Therapy?

Today, all dental schools teach diagnosis of periodontal diseases and their treatment in the early, uncomplicated stages, as well as the basic principles of dental implants.

Therefore, a patient can expect that their family dentist may be the first to recognize and sometimes treat gum disease at its earliest stages. If the progress of the disease is more advanced or associated with complicating factors, consultation with a periodontal specialist is a good idea.

Many patients will find that their dentist uses a team approach to implant therapy, where the general dentist will perform all the prosthetics therapy (placement of abutments and crowns) after the periodontist completes the surgical phase of placing the implants in the jaw.

Are Implants Sensitive to Cold or Hot

No. While in every other respect dental implants may feel just like your own teeth, unlike natural teeth there are no nerves running through the implant, so there is no temperature sensitivity.

What About Seeing My Family Dentist?

You probably have a family or general dentist who is being kept up-to-date with your treatment through correspondence from the periodontist's office. The two professionals work together to ensure you receive all the required treatment in a timely and coordinated fashion throughout the course of therapy. Your periodontist may consult with the dentist regarding changing fillings, new crowns or other restorations, especially in areas of plaque and food catches. After periodontal treatment, you will probably continue to see your periodontist for maintenance, and your dentist for all your other dental needs, including at least a yearly check up.

How Can I Get Rid of Bad Breath Caused by Gum Disease?

While gum diseases are responsible for many cases of bad breath, there are other medical conditions such as digestive problems that can lead to bad breath and should be checked by your physician. However, if the problem is due to gum disease, the most effective means of fighting the embarrassment of bad breath is a consistent and effective oral hygiene routine including brushing twice a day, flossing at least once a day and seeing your dentist on a regular basis.

Mouthwashes and chewing gum can mask the odor of bad breath, but are only short term solutions as they do not address the cause of the problem.

PART IV
Appendix

Finding a Periodontist (Gum Specialist)

Finding a periodontist often begins with a referral from your family dentist, friends or family. Another resource, if you live near a dental school, may be a list of local specialists who are instructors on the school's faculty.

Worldwide, most specialists belong to national or regional specialty organizations that provide a roster of periodontists by geographical area. Listed below is contact information for many periodontal societies throughout the world. This can be helpful, not only for those who reside in the noted countries, but also for frequent travelers who may have a gum related emergency and need expert care.

American Academy of Periodontology: aap.org
　(Note: Each of the 50 States also has its own periodontal society)

Argentina Society of Periodontology: www.saperiodoncia.org.ar

Australian and New Zealand Academy of Periodontists: www.perio.org.au

Austrian Society of Periodontology: www.oegp.at

Belgian Society of Periodontology: www.parodontologie.be

Brazilian Society of Periodontology: www.sobrape.org.br

British Society of Periodontology: www.bsperio.org.uk

Chilean Society of Periodontology: www.spch.cl

Colombian Society of Periodontology: www.encolombia.com

Croatian Society of Periodontology: www.croperio.com

Danish Society of Periodontology: periodont.dk

Dutch Society of Periodontology: www.nvvp.org

Egyptian Periodontal Society: periores@hotmail.com

European Federation of Periodontology: www.efp.net

Canadian Academy of Periodontology: www.cda-adc.ca

Finish Society of Periodontology: www.apollonia.fi

French Society of Periodontology and Oral Implantology: www.sfparo.org

Hellenic Society of Periodontology: www.periodontology.gr

Hungarian Society of Periodontology: gera@fok.usn.hu

Hong Kong Society of Periodontology: www.hongkongperio.org

Indian Society of Periodontology: www.ispperio.com

International Academy of Periodontology: www.perioiap.org

Irish Society of Periodontology: email: perio@ireland.com

Israel Periodontal Society: www.perio.org.il

Italian Society of Periodontology: www.sidp.it

Japanese Society of Periodontology: www.perio.jp

Korean Academy of Periodontology: www.kperio.org

Mexican Society of Periodontology: amp.llamosa@gmail.com

Mongolian Association of Periodontology: amp.tesoreroa@gmail.com

Panamanian Society of Periodontology: nara-78@gmail.com

Peruvian Association of Periodontology: docasal@gmail. com

Polish Society of Periodontology: ford@royalcenter.net

Salvadorian Association of Periodontics: www.perioimplantelsalvador.com

Singapore Society of Periodontology: www.perio.org.sg

South Africa Society of Periodontology: www.perio.org.za

Spanish Society of Periodontology and osseointegration: www.sepa.es

Swedish Society of Periodontology: anna.bogren@odontologi.gu.se

Swiss Society of Periodontology: www.parodontologie.ch

Academy of Periodontology r.o.c. (Taiwan) email: aproc@ms23.hinet.net

Turkish Society of Periodontology: www.turkperio.org

Index

Note to readers of the e-edition: Page numbers are only relevant in the printed edition.

G

Genetic profiling, 56

General dentist's role

in implant therapy, 130

maintenance care, 140

periodontal treatment, 149

Gingiva (gum), 29

Gingivectomy, 105

Gingivitis, 35

Gingivoplasty,105

Grafts, see periodontal surgery

Grinding, see bruxism

Growths, gum, 46

Gum

boil, see abscess

color, changes in, 45

disease, see periodontal diseases

growths, 46

injuries, 42

line, movement after surgery, 116

recession, 38

replacement grafts, 112

swollen, 45

Gummy smile, 113

Gums, 29

H

Halitosis, see bad breath

Harris, Chapin, 21

Hayden, Horace, 21

Healing, the process, 95

Hippocrates, 17

History, dental and medical, 54

History, of man's gum problems, 16

Hygienist, dental, 94, 139

Host response, 34

Hunter, John, 19

I

Implants, see dental implants

Incisors, 27

Initial therapy, 92

Injuries, to gum tissue, 42

Insurance, dental, 144

L

Laughing gas, see nitrous oxide

M

Maintenance, 138

Malocclusion, 95

Medical conditions

influence of periodontal disease, 62

limitations on periodontal care, 118

limitations on implant care, 133

Medications

as alternative to surgery, 119

before surgery, 104

effect on gums, 45

limitations on surgery, 118

Membranes, 110

Mobility of teeth, 58

Molars, 27

Mouth rinses, 88

Ignore Your Teeth and They'll Go Away

Muscle spasms and TMJ, 96, 98

T

V

W

X

About the Author

Dr. Sheldon Dov Sydney has been a practicing gum specialist (periodontist) and educator for over thirty-five years. He is Certified by the American Board of Periodontology and Clinical Associate Professor of Periodontics at the University of Maryland School of Dentistry. Dr. Sydney is former Chief Resident at Emory University, Atlanta, Georgia and President of The Maryland Association of Periodontists. He is also one of the first periodontists in the world to lead a hospital-based department devoted to the relationship between periodontal disease and general body health.

In addition to authoring four editions of *Ignore Your Teeth And They'll Go Away, The Complete Guide to Gum Disease*, Dr. Sydney's original scientific articles have been published in the profession's leading periodicals, and he is a three-time recipient of dentistry's most respected international journalism awards. Dr. Sydney, a well-known presenter at dentistry's most widely attended scientific congresses, has lectured to colleagues and students in more than 20 countries worldwide.

His contributions to dentistry have earned him fellowships in the profession's esteemed honor societies including both the American and the International Colleges of Dentists.

Notes